tPA
FOR
STROKE

tPA

FOR

STROKE

THE STORY OF
A CONTROVERSIAL DRUG

JUSTIN A. ZIVIN, M.D., PH.D

JOHN GALBRAITH SIMMONS

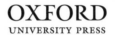
OXFORD
UNIVERSITY PRESS

2011

OXFORD
UNIVERSITY PRESS

Oxford University Press, Inc., publishes works that further
Oxford University's objective of excellence
in research, scholarship, and education.

Oxford   New York
Auckland   Cape Town   Dar es Salaam   Hong Kong   Karachi
Kuala Lumpur   Madrid   Melbourne   Mexico City   Nairobi
New Delhi   Shanghai   Taipei   Toronto

With offices in
Argentina   Austria   Brazil   Chile   Czech Republic   France   Greece
Guatemala   Hungary   Italy   Japan   Poland   Portugal   Singapore
South Korea   Switzerland   Thailand   Turkey   Ukraine   Vietnam

Published by Oxford University Press, Inc.
198 Madison Avenue, New York, New York 10016
www.oup.com

Library of Congress Cataloging-in-Publication Data

Zivin, Justin A.
tPA for stroke : the story of a controversial drug/Justin A. Zivin, John Galbraith Simmons.
p. ; cm.
Includes bibliographical references and index.
ISBN 978-0-19-539392-7
1. Cerebrovascular disease—Chemotherapy—History. 2. Tissue plasminogen activator—Therapeutic
use—History. I. Simmons, John G., 1949–II. Title.
[DNLM: 1. Stroke—drug therapy. 2. Stroke—history. 3. Fibrinolytic Agents—therapeutic use. 4. Tissue
Plasminogen Activator—history. 5. Tissue Plasminogen Activator—therapeutic use. WL 355 Z635t 2011]
RC388.5.Z58 2011
616.8'106—dc22

2010013593

1 3 5 7 9 8 6 4 2

Printed in the United States of America
on acid-free paper

To my wife Reni,
the person who saved one more life than I did
— JAZ

To Jocelyne,
as ever
— JGS

Acknowledgments

*T*he endeavor to bring tPA to bear on acute stroke owes to the dedicated work of a large number of investigators, and in some measure we are indebted to them all. For this book the physicians and scientists we talked with are listed on pages 153-157, and to each of them we wish to offer our thanks and appreciation.

The story of tPA has always been international in scope, and we appreciate the help of Désiré Collen and his associates, whose groundbreaking research inspired researchers worldwide. In the United States we acknowledge all those who participated in the National Institute of Neurological Disorders (NINDS) rt-PA Stroke Study. At a distance of more than 15 years, their collective endeavor constitutes a landmark in making stroke a treatable disorder and a key event in the history of medicine. Among the NINDS researchers, for our story we extend particular thanks to William G. Barson, Joseph P. Broderick, Thomas G. Brott, J. Donald Easton, James C. Grotta, Steven H. Horowitz, Steven R. Levine, Patrick D. Lyden, John R. Marler, Barbara C. Tilley, Michael D. Walker, and K. M. A. Welch.

We would also like to acknowledge the help of Werner Hacke and Markku Kaste, both closely associated with the European Cooperative Acute Stroke Study (ECASS). Our thanks also to Fedor Bachman, Alastair Buchan, Vladimir Hachinski, Kennedy Lees, Didier Leys, Peter Sandercock, and Takenori Yamaguchi.

At Genentech, where work to develop tPA involved some of the best minds in biotech, we thank especially Diane Pennica and also William F. Bennett and Elliott Grossbard.

We are also immensely grateful to Julie Jensen, Don Mead, and Boris Vern for sharing their stories. Our thanks extend to their relatives and colleagues, whose names may be found at the head of the notes to chapters in which they appear, and in this regard, too, we underscore our thanks to Ray Crawford and to Eugene Locken.

At Oxford University Press Sarah Harrington's attention and sensitivity, both to the larger story and to its obscure details, has been of immense help. We thank Susan Lee for helping us meet deadlines and Susan Fensten in efforts to reach a broader audience. Our thanks also to Mark Bowes, who helped bring us together, and to our agent at Writers House, Al Zuckerman.

*** ***

I would like to extend personal thanks to the NINDS investigators, to colleagues at the National Institutes of Health, and to all the investigators who have worked with me over the years. I am especially grateful to my mentors, David Drachman and the late Doug Waud. My thanks too to Marc Fisher and, for frank and helpful comments, to Brett C. Meyer and Mike Roizen. My students at the University of California, San Diego, provided exemplary feedback. I am also grateful to to my daughters Kara and Leslie, both for putting up with me and for reading the book and providing helpful advice.

— J.A.Z.

Let me underscore my gratitude to all those—patients, researchers, and physicians — whom I had the privilege to meet and interview during the extended gestation of this book. Several people provided narrative keys that were more valuable than they could know, among whom I must cite Dan Rifkin and Jeff Saver. For providing candid insights into the advancing situation in emergency medicine I thank Andy Jagoda and Yu-Feng Yvonne Chan at Mount Sinai Medical Center in New York, and Jonathan Edlow at Harvard University. Marcia Stone provided expertise for a key discussion; my brother Garner Simmons and my son Clayton Simmons provided much help throughout, and late-stage advice from Donald-Nicholson Smith was critical. Ben Patrusky, executive director of the Council for the Advancement of Science Writing and formerly with the American Heart Association, recognized the potential for a book about acute stroke, and his encouragement and perspective were more than helpful.

— J.G.S.

Contents

To the Reader

*S*troke is a terrifying and all-too-common event that no one seems much concerned about—until it happens. The third leading cause of death after heart attack and all cancers combined, it is lethal in nearly 3 in 10 cases. But for many more, stroke is a crippling disease. It destroys brains and paralyzes bodies. It robs people of the ability to walk, talk, feed themselves, and conduct the activities of daily life. Worldwide, the annual toll of permanent disability from stroke is some *5 million* people.

The great majority of strokes—more than 8 in 10—are due to blocked or clogged blood vessels that starve brain tissue, which then deteriorates and dies. Most patients with such strokes would benefit from the "clot-busting" medicine known as *tissue plasminogen activator*, or tPA. If given in a timely way—within 4.5 hours after symptoms appear—this drug can prevent or substantially reduce the wide variety of cognitive and physical deficits that a stroke inflicts.

But if you suffer a stroke today, depending on where you go for treatment and how fast you get there, your chances of getting the drug probably range from not very likely to nearly negligible. Although approved by the Food and Drug Administration (FDA) in 1996 and endorsed by major medical organizations, the use of tPA for stroke is controversial—for many reasons, all worth discussing but none of them very good. As one consequence, knowledge that tPA even exists is not widespread among the general public. While a majority of stroke patients would in principle be eligible for tPA, in fact the drug has been restricted to a fortunate few.

"I label this a national tragedy or a national embarrassment," says Mark J. Alberts, professor of neurology at the Feinberg School of Medicine at Northwestern University. "I know of no disease that is as common or as serious as stroke and where you basically have one therapy and it's only used in 3% to 4% of patients. That's like saying you only treat 3% to 4% of patients with bacterial pneumonia with antibiotics."

Nothing about these low numbers argues for inevitability. They can change. That is why we are writing this book.

In the chapters that follow we explain what tPA is and investigate why it has been so little used. Broadly, stroke victims have been hamstrung between neurologists not accustomed to caring for emergencies and emergency doctors fearful of treating a brain disorder. For various reasons, decent and well-intentioned leaders of stroke neurology fomented initial opposition to and skepticism of tPA that abided even after they themselves changed their minds about the drug. Persistent opponents of tPA in emergency medicine, though their ranks have diminished, continue to undermine efforts to reach more patients and save more brains. In the course of our story, we will examine those quarrels and address them from a scientific perspective. A persistent and unfortunate tension between science and medicine is a recurring theme in the story of tPA for stroke.

To raise awareness of tPA, to get the word out, is our principal objective. For many diseases, one expects that doctors know a great deal about any given treatment and their patients, correspondingly little. With stroke and tPA, however, an excess of such "asymmetrical knowledge" is unfortunate; ignorance on the part of patients is a decided negative. So we reach out to a wide and general audience in the hope of redressing the balance. Potential stroke victims and their friends and families need to know the symptoms of stroke. They should be aware that stroke is an acute emergency and of the simple rule: call 911. But they also need to know about tPA, to realize that most patients are eligible to receive it if they seek help immediately—that, in short, "time is brain." By explaining why this is so, and providing the facts about the trials and controversies that have surrounded the drug for more than a decade, we hope to turn people's passive knowledge into an active grasp of how tPA works and why they need to know about it. That kind of knowledge might one day help them, or family members and friends, avoid the kind of severe disability that can too often be characterized as "a fate worse than death." Quite fortunately, tPA was one of the first and most successful drugs to emerge from the so-called "biotech" revolution. Its intriguing history has much to say about how contemporary medicine works—or fails to work—and the pursuit of useful drugs.

A word concerning our collaboration is in order. One of us (Zivin) was one of the earliest investigators of tPA for stroke. He performed some of the first experiments, participated in the clinical trials, and became a proponent favoring wide implementation of the drug after its 1996 approval by the FDA. But he does not set out here to write a personal memoir; rather, this book has the broader aim of telling the story of what is generally acknowledged as the most controversial drug ever used in neurology. Accordingly, we have adopted a narrative approach that makes room for a variety of voices and viewpoints, weaving the principal discoveries, experiments, and trials into a larger narrative. To that end, it should be emphasized, our final product is a line-by-line collaboration. Zivin told the initial story and drew upon 30 years of work in research and clinical neurology to provide details that Simmons, who writes about both contemporary issues and the history of science and medicine, made independent efforts to verify or falsify. The stroke literature, together with inputs from several dozen neurologists, emergency medicine physicians, statisticians, and others, helped to cast and detail the story that finally emerged. Its rough textures and sometimes strident tones reflect the conflicting views and human interactions that are ever-present in important scientific and medical discoveries. In a postscript, Zivin details his scientific disputes and conflicts concerning the now-famous trials that led to FDA approval of tPA for stroke.

Overall, we follow a simple plan. Part 1 tells about stroke and the discovery of tPA, and how it was found to be potentially useful and then tested in people. Part 2 discusses the controversies and issues that arose after FDA approval and that continue to restrict its use today. Because tPA is one of the most powerful drugs ever developed, this is also emphatically a story about medicine in our time, replete with perplexing paradoxes for health care, frustration for doctors and, when underused, bad outcomes for patients. Although repeatedly shown to be cost-effective, tPA has been underused in part due to inadequate compensation for both physicians and hospitals. Today, as its promise moves somewhat closer to fulfillment, failure to give the drug when appropriate has raised troublesome and disturbing legal issues. Finally, tPA has started to advance internationally in ways that deserve attention. Throughout we make an effort to stay close to the real-world consequences of inaction.

Fifteen years after it was approved, tPA remains the only useful treatment for acute stroke. In years to come we may hope for new drugs and devices, but universal recognition of the telltale symptoms of stroke and the crucial importance of seeking rapid treatment are likely to remain constant goals. For the present, tPA is indispensable, as more and more doctors have come to recognize. Among patients themselves, tPA should help relieve some of the pessimism, denial, and resignation associated with stroke, but so far it has barely scratched the surface.

Part | 1

Discovery

Code Stroke on Market Street | 1

For Julie Milanese, after weeks of long hours and grueling travel, another work-day ended late. A meeting ran over schedule and quarter-past five found her still at her desk, leaving somebody a phone message. Then, while typing a final e-mail, she registered surprise because suddenly her left arm did not seem to belong to her body.

This disconcerting impression quickly vanished. She took a breath and looked again. Her arm was there. She wondered if colleagues were playing tricks on her, slipping a rubber prosthesis onto her desk. But Halloween was still a month away.

"Julie, are you all right?"

Sitting next to her, Steve Kondonijakos had heard her talking on the phone.

"Yes, I'm fine. Why?"

It was September 30, 2004. At 26, Julie was an associate media director with 4 years in interactive advertising at Organic, Inc., a digital marketing firm on Market Street in San Francisco. She was Italianate, pretty and bright, serious and self-possessed, slender and blue-eyed with an oval face and a cascade of dark brown curls. Recently she had gotten engaged.

Now the left side of her body just stopped working. Her arm flopped uselessly on the desk.

"You're slurring," said Steve.

She did not hear the incompetence in her voice, yet struggled when she tried to reply.

Steve exchanged a glance with Eric, a colleague. Eric had also heard the out-of-synch voice and experienced the same distress. In speech and appearance she seemed so wrong. Julie was alarmingly not Julie.

Fear and anxiety rapidly suffused the workplace. Steve and Eric sought the attention of Julie's sister, Erica. She worked at Organic, too, just cubicles away. Four years younger than Julie, Erica was considered more ready to laugh, more cheerful by nature—yet she was a worrier. No sooner had she asked, "What's wrong?" than she noticed Julie's hand, uncontrolled and weirdly curled.

Nobody said "stroke." Steve, whose grandfather had suffered one a dozen years earlier, refrained from alarming Erica, and kept quiet. But Erica herself recognized something about her sister's gnarled hand. She was reminded of their grandmother, who had been confined to a wheelchair for the past 14 years. Same hand. Erica didn't say "stroke," either.

Word spread. Everybody in the office gathered around Julie's desk. Each voiced a different solution. Perhaps it was epilepsy, fatigue, or low blood sugar. Julie herself did not seem too distressed. She was calm and her arm flopped and her words came out distorted. She was not in pain.

Stroke is an ancient disease and inspires fear and trembling. That the word went unsaid in the offices of Organic that afternoon was in its own way tragic, reflecting a common and collective reluctance to face one of life's most danger-ous events. Stroke newly afflicts almost three quarters of a million people each year in the United States alone.

Yet in Julie's case, a quickened sense of mortal danger prevailed over inevita-ble appeals to let's-wait-and-see. Spurred by Erica's sense of urgency, co-workers called 911.

Almost one person in four who suffers a stroke will die from it in short order. Nearly the same number totally recovers. But the bulbous 50% in the middle suffer emotional agony and physical disability in the weeks, months, and years that follow. Survivors may be paralyzed, unable walk, to talk, and to think. Brief strokes, called transient ischemic attacks (TIAs), are by definition harmless, but they often presage the real thing. A stroke can be accurately called a "brain attack," a term that conveys its similarity to heart attack. Both are due to clogged or broken blood vessels.

Unlike heart attack, though, for which a raft of treatments became available in the last three decades of the 20th century, stroke remained into the 1990s a dread event for which doctors could do nothing. Physicians could no more do anything useful for a patient with a stroke-in-progress, whose brain tissue was beginning to decay, than a police officer could stop a car wreck during a collision. Treating a stroke was just as futile 20 years ago as it was 2,000 years ago. Neurologist David Drachman, who trained in the 1950s, remembers, "It was sort of believed there was no point in doing something about it. You merely hoped there would be restitution of function when other areas of the brain took over. Once there was a stroke, that was just about it."

Rehabilitation through physical therapy might come in the wake of a stroke, but for many victims it does little good. Useful for patient morale, stroke rehab is a substantial industry unto itself. But truth to tell, recovery is virtually complete for most patients by the end of the first month. This fact is largely concealed in medicine today, a case of good intentions furthering an ostrich-like stance that, when it comes to stroke, has been prevalent and obstinate.

History provides abundant examples of famous people brought down by stroke, and also of the associated stigma that provokes lies and concealment. In 1919 President Woodrow Wilson suffered a series of strokes that left him half-paralyzed, blind in one eye, and mentally unable to govern, with the result that the United States was without an effective chief executive for 18 world-shaping months, until 1921. For decades afterward the extent of Wilson's disability was kept secret.

Similarly, the deteriorating physical condition of Franklin Delano Roosevelt was hidden from the world during World War II. The president suffered from cardiovascular disease and morbidly high blood pressure—ranging up to 260/150—that placed him just outside death's door when he went to negotiate the post-war world at Yalta in February 1945. After he suddenly died 2 months later, his doctor, Admiral Ross McIntire, continued to prevaricate. He said Roosevelt had been in excellent health and that apoplexy (an old-fashioned term for stroke) "came out of the clear sky."

Everybody in Julie's department at work took notice. At least a half-dozen friendly and concerned employees swarmed around her. One co-worker, Heather, quickly saw that the problem must be Julie's brain. She kept calm, spoke quietly, and offered water but Julie was unable to drink. Could she stick out her tongue? Kneeling beside her, Heather squeezed Julie's left foot.

"Can you feel this?"

"Feel what?" asked Julie.

An emergency medical team was on its way. Meanwhile, Julie could stand by herself but not walk. Humor had deserted her but she had no sense of panic or even particular urgency despite the onset of paralysis. She was not in pain. Co-workers wheeled her into the lobby and eased her onto a couch. Heather comforted her with words about her future and her engagement to Doug. Not 10 minutes passed before the ambulance arrived.

Ray Crawford, a pleasant, mustachioed former fireman, was the paramedic who led the emergency medicine team. He kneeled beside Julie.

"Thanks for coming," she said. "But I feel fine. I'm not exactly sure why you're here but thanks for taking care of me."

Julie saw Ray was in his mid- to late forties, of average build with reddish-blond hair. She did not see his mustache. Where his face ought to be she saw only a blur. The same was true, in fact, of her co-workers. She knew each by voice and physical outline, but just now she could not make out their faces. Everyone, it seemed, was faceless.

"Let's take you in," said Ray gently, betraying no alarm, "just in case."

In Ray's own mind, as they placed Julie on the gurney and rolled her outside and lifted her into the ambulance, there was no doubt. Her slurred speech and failed left side, not to say insouciance and bewilderment, made this case transparent.

"I am very concerned," he said, taking Erica aside. "It looks like your sister had or is having a stroke."

Erica felt rising panic, but Ray warned her to keep a poker face. A spike in Julie's blood pressure would not help. Erica must bluff and stay calm. "The only one that needs to know the reality," said Ray, "is you."

Until this moment, Julie had been in superb physical shape. Her weight and heart health were exemplary. She ran marathons, cycled, and participated in tri-athlons. Last week she had played baseball. Yoga every day. Low blood pressure. She never smoked.

At 5:30 that afternoon, September 30, 2004, Julie Milanese looked liked a textbook case, in a young person, of a serious, potentially massive, and evolving stroke.

A stroke happens, in most cases, when blood flow to some part of the brain slows or stops. A broken blood vessel, which causes bleeding into the brain, can also cause stroke. But about 87% of the time, the precipitating cause is a clog due to narrowed vessels or a clot. Blood stalls. Within minutes, when oxygen and nutrients cannot reach brain cells, tissue starts to feel deprived. As that happens, brain circuits malfunction and ischemic stroke occurs. The various symptoms are all the more treacherous for being painless: dizziness, vertigo, vision loss or troubled speech, numbness, and inability to move the face or an arm or leg, usually localized to one side of the body. Julie that afternoon was a perfect example.

Many people imagine stroke as a disordered but brief final blow closing out the lives of geriatric patients, making Julie, at 26, a rare exception. That is a misapprehension. Risk of dying from a stroke does indeed spike after age 60, but that is not old by today's standards. Each year, about 3 in 10 people who suffer stroke are under 65. Strokes in young people are unexpected but they happen. Strokes can afflict at any age; even babies can suffer strokes.

Thinking of stroke as an old person's disease and final fatal meltdown is one of the pervasive beliefs and impressions that makes treating stroke as a genuine emergency so terribly problematic. For some years in the recent past the number of strokes actually declined, probably because many were due to high blood pressure, successfully treatable from the 1960s. Grandfathers, grandmothers, and aging mothers and fathers are always being felled by strokes. Indeed, it has only recently become widely viewed as an emergency. Among Julie's co-workers that afternoon were those who suggested she might best take a nap.

Still the number-three killer in most of the industrialized world, strokes afflict more than 750,000 people each year in the United States alone—a new case every 45 seconds. Stroke is also the leading cause of adult disability. In young adults, though less deadly overall than in older people, stroke can be unsparing and put victims, if not promptly treated, at high risk of disability. One study from Israel, published in 1996, showed that that 87% of some 253 ischemic stroke victims, aged 17 to 49, were left with a disability; in 19% disability was moderate, and in 19%, severe. For young people as well as old, stroke can be a permanent health catastrophe.

Ray Crawford in principle had no choice. California rules laid down that, unless patients make other demands, paramedics must take them to the nearest emergency facility. Paramedics are paid to transport, not diagnose. But that late afternoon on Market Street, Ray did exactly that. He diagnosed.

Ray made a point of treating patients the way he would his own family. Before taking off in the ambulance, he told Erica quietly, "Listen, if this were me, I would take her to UCSF," the University of California, San Francisco Medical Center. It was not the nearest emergency department. Two others, at San Francisco General and at St. Francis Memorial Hospital, were closer, each just a mile and a few minutes away. UCSF was 5 miles away—and this was rush hour.

"We're going to have to pass almost every hospital in the city to get there."

But Ray knew UCSF was obtaining official certification as a stroke center. Whatever that meant, he knew that at least there would be a neurologist on duty who could ensure that Julie received tPA if she was eligible—and it looked like she was. This would not be the case elsewhere. The nearer emergency rooms might not even risk treating Julie but transfer her, losing precious time. Ray knew that lost minutes cost huge numbers of brain cells. Erica deferred to his advice.

Once Julie was in the rig and they were off, Ray alerted the hospital—calling twice, then a third time. He emphasized the woman was young and a candidate for therapy. To prime the stroke team, he adopted an urgent tone. Ray had a philosophy about this. "You know which cases to jump up on your pedestal and bark about, and which to let slide. You don't get your panties in a knot. You don't get upset about non-acute ones."

The ambulance ride Ray deemed worth taking would last some 20-odd minutes. Following a simple protocol, he reassessed Julie's overall appearance, administered oxygen, inserted two IVs—one for saline, another in case she would get tPA—and monitored her heart and blood pressure. As the ambulance howled its way through the jammed rush-hour canyon, Julie submitted to all this, feeling irritated. Away from the non-faces of co-workers, she had a moment of self-reflection. She knew her sister was somewhere. But Erica seemed far away and that was not right. "For goodness' sake," she thought, "I'm lying here in the back of the ambulance. I'm starting to go paralyzed and she hasn't said a word to me. I can't believe that."

In fact, Erica was up front with the driver, where Ray had made sure she was not near Julie. Maybe she should remain collected, but she was not. If waiting for the medics had been the worst 10 minutes of Erica's life, this drive to the hospital was the next most distressing 25. Yet she managed to call their father, Rick, who was at work, about half an hour away. Then Doug, Julie's fiancé. He was closer. But their mother, Teri, was in San Bruno, a good 12 miles distant and, with traffic, nearly an hour away. They would all meet at the hospital.

Behind her, she could hear Julie mumbling incoherently, unable to make sense, her left side paralyzed.

Why clots form, disrupting circulation to the brain and causing symptoms such as paralysis, often remains unknown. Certainly, blood clot formation is an essential repair mechanism for complex organisms. But ultimately clots are unwelcome products of various pathological conditions afflicting the lungs, heart, and other organs—including the brain. A few simple words describe them. A *thrombus* is simply a clot located within a blood vessel, further qualified by where it happens. Thus, *cerebral thrombosis* is the most common type of stroke: a thrombus in an artery that nourishes the brain. An *embolus*—as in Julie's case, it turned out—is a broken-off portion of a thrombus that travels through the blood and becomes lodged in a distant vessel.

How blood coagulates and clots form were for centuries substantially a mystery. Old explanations, such as heat and exposure to air, were clearly inadequate. Only in 1905 did a Russian-born German scientist, Paul Morawitz, propose what became the "classic" theory. It is fairly easy to understand. All blood clots, including those that cause ischemic stroke, arise through an enzymatic chain reaction. Enzymes, the type of proteins that dramatically speed up every sort of physiological reaction, are responsible.* Some injury or break in a blood vessel ultimately calls into play a specific enzyme known as *thrombokinase*, which connects with and modifies a precursor molecule named *prothrombin*. The result is *thrombin*, a clot-promoting substance that presides over the conversion of *fibrinogen*, another precursor, into *fibrin*, the essential fibrous-like scaffolding of clots.

Much research has elaborated the chemistry over the course of the past century, but this four-factor recipe for blood coagulation was essentially correct. To put it simply, blood coagulates in a stepwise fashion to plug and protect the integrity of the vascular system. However, when such a plug lodges in a place where it causes harm, thrombosis is the result.

If clots are necessary for survival, equally important are the chemical reactions that dissolve them. This system in its fundamentals also comprises a straightforward series of enzymatic steps. An "activator" converts idle *plasminogen* to *plasmin*, which is a powerful fibrin-dissolving—hence clot-destroying—enzyme. Tissue plasminogen activator (tPA) is the molecule in question. It has the special property of acting upon plasminogen only in the presence of fibrin—only where there is a clot. A whole sub-discipline, known as fibrinolytics, has developed to investigate the intricacies of clot dissolution.

A failure of the fibrinolytic system—if a clot is too big for the body's own tPA to readily and promptly dissolve it—can lead to thrombosis and, in Julie's case, to a stroke. Here is where tPA as a drug comes into play.

The admitting physician at UCSF also had no discernible face; she too was a featureless blur. But Julie heard her. She greeted her with a brisk, "Ma'am, do you know what's happening to you?"

"Actually, I think I had a stroke."

"No, Ma'am. You *are having* a stroke."

Julie had always conceived of stroke as a lightning-like moment.

"We're going to put you on the CT scan to determine what kind of stroke you're having."

Julie remained compliant even as she recognized paralysis; she was no longer aware of the left side of her body. She told herself she could panic or else try to relax and let other people take care of her. Besides, in the ambulance powerful fatigue had settled upon her together with the alarming idea she

---

*We avoid chemical terminology where we can, but a few words such as *enzymes* require clarification. An enzyme *precursor* is present but latent until an *activator* converts it to its rapid-acting form. There also exist corresponding molecular inhibitors that work to slow and stop enzymatic activity.

might sleep forever if she closed her eyes. That thought made her strive to stay awake. She did not complain as she was rolled into an elevator and taken to the radiology suite.

With computerized tomography, or CT, doctors can quickly visualize the brain's soft tissue, invisible on traditional X-ray, to rule out a bleeding stroke. As she was wheeled toward the machine, Julie could hear the nurse's strident voice, encountering another patient in the scanner.

"This woman's having a stroke. Get him off. She has to get on now. Take him off *now*."

Downstairs in the emergency room, while Julie was being scanned, Doug Jensen, Julie's fiancé, arrived. Soon after, her father, Rick Milanese, came in. Erica greeted him in tears and Doug said to him, "Time is of the essence."

That was what the emergency room doctor told them. The stroke was happening in a major artery of Julie's brain, which explained why she was losing mobility on the left side. As next of kin, Rick and Erica might need to make the decision as to tPA. Assuming no bleeding, she was a good candidate, young and otherwise healthy. But the risks, so they were told, included death. Julie was not improving; her symptoms were worsening and whether she would be competent to make a decision herself was unclear.

Shoehorned into a tiny office, they were left to discuss the tPA option among themselves.

"The clock is ticking," said Rick.

As a family, the Milaneses belonged to San Francisco's computer generation and the dotcom world. They were also a traditional intact family, with dinner on the table at 6:30. Bearded and thoughtful, Rick was usually cheerful and confident, but not now. He worked in computer storage, not brain preservation. Risk of death sucked the wind out of them all.

But their consent turned out to be unnecessary. Julie, brought back to the emergency room after the scan, was met by a nurse, who spoke very fast. Doctors had examined the pictures. "You're having a stroke, an embolic stroke. You have a clot lodged in your right carotid artery. Now we have this drug that could save your life." She added quickly, "But there is a potential it could kill you."

Julie slurred, "Okay, but it could help?"

"Yes, there's a possibility it could help you," said the nurse.

Julie signed the paperwork with her unaffected right hand.

tPA is one of the most controversial drugs ever. That it was one of the first products of the biotech revolution proved to be not a mark in its favor but a reason for suspicion. It was originally used and approved in the 1980s for heart attack, and what seemed like its relatively high cost provided grist for stories of

Big Pharma greed and unethical collusion between doctors and drug marketers. When it came to stroke, such suspicion bolstered obstinate skepticism and disbelief even while, time and again, research continued to show that the drug works.

To be effective, tPA for stroke must be administered within 4.5 hours after symptoms start—and in any event, the sooner the better. (Three hours was for a long time the limit but recent trials extended that time window, and other efforts to further lengthen time-to-treatment may one day succeed.) Recognizing that a stroke victim requires urgent treatment and rapid transport to the nearest emergency room are both essential. But as matters currently stand, neither of these measures guarantees tPA for eligible patients. Although the protocol, or set of rules for administering tPA, is fairly simple, it is often not used or even offered.

Ideological barriers have retarded use of tPA over the past decade and a half. During that time many thousands of brains have been unnecessarily damaged. No other drug has been developed in the interim that works as well; many more have been shown to fail. Nevertheless, the debates among neurologists around tPA for stroke between 1996 and 2002 continue to affect treatment today, years later. Hostility from emergency physicians, especially from some of the leaders in the field of emergency medicine, has created reluctance to learn about and use tPA.

At 6:45 that evening, about 90 minutes after her first symptoms, the emergency room staff injected Julie with tPA through the IV that Ray Crawford had started in the ambulance 40 minutes earlier. tPA is freshly mixed for each patient, and the dose is based on body weight. Apart from that, it is a simple injection and intravenous drip.

The neurologist on the stroke team, Vineeta Singh, a calm critical care specialist, first evaluated Julie while the tPA was dripping. By now, her patient was not really aware of what was happening.

"What's the matter with you?" she asked Julie.

"My head. My head is hurting." Julie gestured with her right hand while her left arm flailed out of control. She did not seem to notice it.

Nor was Julie concerned about her symptoms. She asked when she could return to yoga and her exercise regime. When could she go home?

"We'll talk about that tomorrow," said Dr. Singh. "Tonight you are staying in the hospital."

Teri, Julie's mother, was the last family member to arrive. Meeting her outside the emergency room, Rick told her the diagnosis. She broke down and cried. After holding each other a long while, they went inside to find Erica and Doug. Together they went to see Julie about 7:15 that evening. When she saw Teri, Julie cried for the first and only time.

"I'm sorry I made you worry," she managed.

On the left side, with no mobility or motion, her face drooped. Julie knew something important was happening but had no insight into the gravity of her situation and was barely aware of her surroundings. When she saw Doug, she attempted a smile and asked if he still wanted to marry her. He said yes and told her he loved her.

Doug and Julie had met some 6 years ago, just as she finished college. Unlike Julie, he had not grown up in San Francisco but in London; his family had lived in Iran but fled not long after he was born, when in 1979 the Shah was overthrown. Doug had deep-set brown eyes, a high forehead, and a softly shaped lantern jaw. He and Julie carried on a long-distance relationship for a couple of years before moving in together. They lived in the Richmond district of San Francisco, just a few blocks away. He had proposed to her 3 months ago, in June.

Now, with Rick standing over his daughter, Doug leaned across and took his hand.

For family members and those close to stroke victims, dire prospects can bring fortitude. People take on emotionally more than any human being ought to bear. Death is a quartile likelihood, helplessness and loss of personhood another sword of Damocles. To the sudden and drastic symptoms of diminished brain are superadded total uncertainty as to outcome.

"This makes no difference," said Doug to Rick. "I'm in it for the duration."

The Milaneses and Doug followed Julie up to the neuro-intensive care unit, or NICU. They gathered around while, from time to time, a nurse came in to test her left side, running a finger along her foot in an effort to elicit the Babinski reflex. Doug too tried to stimulate that side. He caressed her legs and arms with the tips of his fingers.

Rick, Teri, Erica, and Doug stayed in the NICU until forced to leave at 11:30 that night. Julie was calm. Nurses came by every hour to monitor her neural signs. Her blood pressure was under invasive scrutiny by another needle in her arm. At intervals more blood was drawn for laboratory studies.

For now, she was paralyzed.

Clot-buster: The Natural History | 2

Alfons Billau—friends call him Fons—once made two trips to the city of Rotterdam in a single day, doubling back to Belgium so he could pick up and deliver vials of a new and untested drug. At a medical conference reception on April 21, 1981, Fons, a cell biologist, had met a physician and friend, Willem Weimar, who said that one of his patients had just shown up in the emergency ward. She was suffering from a grave complication in the wake of a kidney transplant: a thrombus in the principal vein leading from the graft. The huge blood clot was visible on X-ray, floating within the inferior vena cava, the big vein that receives blood from the major organs and the lower limbs. It obstructed circulation. If nothing was done, the patient, a 30-year-old woman, could be expected to lose her new kidney and, in addition, she ran no small risk for heart attack and stroke. Her condition was life-threatening. But so far as Weimar knew, there was nothing he could do.

"Ever heard of HEPA?" asked Fons. The letters stood for *human extrinsic plasminogen activator*. Weimar had not. So far he had treated the woman with cortisone and started her on anticoagulant therapy, both to no avail.

HEPA was a potent substance that seemed to dissolve clots without increasing the risk of bleeding. Extracted from an unexpected source—cancer cells—the substance had been recently purified. Was it worth trying on this patient? Weimar thought that it was.

So Fons returned to Leuven. He knew about HEPA in the first place only because he had helped biochemist Désiré Collen grow the cells that produced it. He remembered the day when the Belgian scientist suddenly showed up with a flask of the cells, just arrived from the United States, requesting he grow them in his laboratory. He obliged. Now from Collen, who was only too happy to provide it, he collected a vial of the purified stuff they were calling HEPA, packed it in ice, and drove back to Rotterdam.

When he injected his patient, Weimar wrote later, "The clot completely dissolved." There were no side effects. The patient recovered. "We wrote a *Lancet* paper and Désiré became famous," he recalled laconically. Twenty-eight years later the patient was still alive. HEPA was soon recognized to be identical to endogenous tPA—the body's own clot-dissolving molecule.

But Fons Billau provided the genuinely salient comment. "The case was reminiscent," he wrote, "of the first evidence for the clinical effectiveness of penicillin."

It was an apt and revealing comparison in terms of science, medicine, and social context. Penicillin, the original wonder drug, and tPA are similar in multiple ways and also present intriguing contrasts.

The two are comparable in power though exclusive as to realm of action. Penicillin obliterates bacteria; tPA destroys blood clots. Used to treat a host of infectious diseases, penicillin and later derivatives represent a pivotal turning point in modern medicine. Although tPA has a narrower range of applications, it is effective in two of the most common lethal disorders in today's world: heart attack and stroke.

Why do these drugs work? Both products exist in nature, but one is more perplexing than the other. Seventy years after its discovery, nobody knows why penicillin exists at all. With its ability to break down bacterial cell walls while sparing most people either toxic side effects or allergic reactions, it is best described as a "gift from nature." Manufactured as a drug, resistant strains of bacteria have come to limit its usefulness. By contrast, tPA is an endogenous enzyme, key to a highly evolved clot-dissolving system common though not identical in all mammals; neither resistance nor allergy is an issue.

Scientific parallels are equally fascinating. Both penicillin and tPA derived from investigations into "lysis"—that is, enzymatic dissolution, whether the object to be dissolved is bacteria or blood clots. Alexander Fleming, who discovered penicillin, wrote a brief paper about it in 1929 but was not able to progress to genuine clinical applications. A decade later his neglected article came to the attention of research pathologist Howard Florey and biochemist Ernst Chain, who were working together on a plan to study all natural antibiotics at the beginning of World War II. The need for improved medicines to combat infection was a harsh lesson from the Great War 20 years before. Research alliances forged mainly with U.S. pharmaceutical companies made it possible to quickly purify the bread-mold substance, scale up production, and move it into the real world of clinical medicine. Similarly, tPA arose from research on the fibrinolytic system—yet, by contrast, extraction and purification were conundrums that impeded research for decades. In addition, both drugs had less effective antecedents: sulfa drugs came before penicillin, and streptokinase preceded tPA.

The discovery of both penicillin and tPA involved a mix of happenstance and good science. Fleming first stumbled upon an antibiotic event in a Petri dish that some suspect owed to spores carried into his laboratory from the floor below, where another scientist was collecting various molds. But it required determined research and investment to create a drug of it. Similarly, the discovery of tPA was "decisively influenced by a few serendipitous observations and very simple experiments," wrote Désiré Collen, who explicitly hoped to counter the impression of an orderly progression of experiments. But once recognized for what it was, as with penicillin, a directed research program rapidly brought it to fruition.

But standing in stark contrast to the comparable power and mechanism of action of penicillin and tPA are their historical receptions. Penicillin was the drug that practically defined the therapeutic revolution in the last half of the 20th century. One could scarcely overstate the positive welcome it received in the 1940s. Doctors embraced it without quarrel. With its entry into the clinic during World War II, wrote the late historian of medicine, Roy Porter, it was a clear sign that the "long anticipated therapeutic revolution had...arrived." Charles Fletcher, who administered the first dose of the drug to a human patient, recalled how the old septic wards—those "chambers of horror" for infected patients—disappeared from hospitals. Penicillin was the first in a cavalcade of drug discovery in the larger context of postwar prosperity.

The situation when tPA came on the scene was entirely different. Forty and 50 years after the marketing of penicillin, medicine was a hugely scaled-up enterprise. A revolution in biology and profound advances throughout biochemistry led to a vast expansion of research. These were the scientific motors behind the creation of a sprawling system of health care. And while modern medicine meant longer lives that could be healthier for many, the price tag was high and mounting. Public confidence in medicine, which spiked with the advent of penicillin in the 1940s, had soured and eroded less than half a century later. Sociologist Paul Starr, in *The Social Transformation of American Medicine*, described "the end of a mandate" as beginning in the 1970s. This was true even as treatments for heart attack and acute stroke—the first and third most common cause of death, respectively—were much desired. This tectonic shift in public attitudes, which eventually became part and parcel of the longstanding if not permanent crisis in health care in the United States, provoked ambivalent attitudes toward new drugs. Brought to market for heart attack in the late 1980s, by the time the FDA approved it for stroke in 1996, tPA would by no means encounter a warm reception like penicillin but rather skepticism, suspicion, and initial rejection.

The bare discovery of tPA as a unique substance is usually dated to 1947 and experiments by Danish investigators Tage Astrup and Per M. Permin. Clots that they introduced into slices of tissue from various mammals—oxen, pigs, rabbits, and rats—would lyse, or dissolve. The agent responsible, hypothetically at first, was eventually named tissue plasminogen activator, or tPA. Within a few years this discovery brought about elucidation of the stepwise series of enzyme-controlled events described in Chapter 1. Again, in the presence of a fibrin clot, tPA activates plasminogen, which converts to plasmin to dissolve the dense scaffolding of thrombi and emboli.

Although the system seemed simple enough, nothing proved easy with tPA. Extractability was the first obstacle. Scientists could deduce its activity and eventually test for its presence, but they could not separate tPA from the tissue in which they found it. It resisted purification. Not exactly ghostly, but they could hardly bottle it. At first, nobody seems to have thought much about making a drug out of tPA, but in any event scarcity was a powerful limitation to experimentation—a situation that would long persist. Between the detection of tPA and scientists' ability to experiment with it in purified form, 35 years would elapse—a long walk, one might say, between drinks.

Medicine does not wait on molecules, however. Fibrinolytics research acquired clinical urgency as physicians in the 1940s recognized there were patients with various disorders arising from intravascular clots. Indeed, heart attack was one of them—a disease of increasing incidence and high mortality. If tPA could not be extracted from the various tissues in which it was known to reside, including blood, there were additional possibilities. Enzymes discovered in animals or somewhere in nature might serve as clot dissolvers—if they could only be found. Indeed, another activator of plasminogen, called urokinase, was extracted from urine and also tested as a fibrinolytic agent. Fruitless efforts would be made to discover synthetic chemicals that lysed clots. Most significant was the bacteria-derived agent eventually developed as a drug that would help pave the way for tPA: streptokinase.

Long on promise though imperfect, streptokinase emerged from the laboratory of a prominent microbiologist, William Smith Tillett. In 1933 Tillett had observed—by chance, the historical accounts all emphasize—that adding a strain of streptococcal bacteria to a test tube of clotted blood would liquefy it. He recognized that the bacteria must contain a "lytic factor" that operated on fibrin. Not himself adequately trained for the sort of chemical analysis required, he brought into his laboratory investigators who helped him isolate and purify the "factor" the bacteria exuded. Tillett understood that the bacterial origins of the substance meant it could be cultured in quantity and perhaps had a future as a drug.

These events and experiments all took place, it should be added, in the higher echelons of American medicine. First at Johns Hopkins, then as chief of medicine at New York University School of Medicine, Tillett helped inaugurate a whole school of fibrinolytics research in the United States. Its leader was his student, physician Sol Sherry, first in New York at Bellevue Hospital and later at Washington University in St. Louis. In 1946 Tillett put Sherry in charge of investigating streptokinase for its therapeutic potential. After test-tube experiments came trial efforts with individual patients.

"In 1949, we published the first in vivo demonstration of the lysis of clotted human blood," wrote Sherry of the early experimental work with human patients. Within a year he was using streptokinase to treat conditions in which blood clots accumulated around some organ in the body; tubercular meningitis and hemothorax (blood in the pleural cavity) were two examples.

But from the beginning, Sherry always emphasized his work "was based on its ultimate use in the treatment of acute coronary thrombosis"—then the common term for heart attack, reflecting the belief of many—correct, though not shared by all—that clots were the most prevalent cause.

Streptokinase had a rocky but partly successful career, early and late. Purity was a serious problem at first, making it unsuitable for intravenous administration such as would be essential with heart attack. The pharmaceutical firm Lederle undertook the task of improving it, largely succeeding about 1957. Shortly thereafter, Sherry attracted widespread attention with encouraging results from a pilot study. However, in spite of some success during the 1960s, uncertainties over dosing and concerns about bleeding continued to plague streptokinase. Although cardiologists had become adept at treating heart attack as an emergency and were eager for a thrombolytic, the drug carried such an uncomfortable burden of risk and different protocols that Lederle eventually ran into legal problems. It shut down production, which was subsequently taken up by a European firm.

For stroke, the promise of streptokinase was not lost on neurologists. But when the drug was tested for this purpose during the early 1960s, it failed. A group led by John S. Meyer at Wayne State University performed several studies with outcomes ranging from uncertain, to bad, to worse. In hindsight one can clearly see, among other flaws, that starting patients on the drug up to 3 days after symptoms appeared was far too late. In one cohort of 73 patients, Meyer reported that 13 of 37 patients who received streptokinase died—versus 4 deaths among 36 controls. Outcomes of these trials probably instilled the notion among neurologists that, as the authors of one review article put it in 1977, "[I]t must be concluded that, although theoretically attractive, the employment of thrombolytic therapy in acute cerebral ischemia appears to lack benefit and… may, in fact, be hazardous."

Limitations of streptokinase for heart attack also led to frustration, which, of course, has been one of medicine's defining characteristics for a couple of thousand years. And also a perennial consequence: a new theory without foundation. For a moment in the latter half of the 20th century, many cardiologists returned to the 19th century as doctors began to wonder if clot-busting therapy for heart attack was of any use in the first place.

In the 1840s Rudolph Virchow first advanced the terms *thrombus* and *embolus* to describe the clots inside blood vessels. He explicitly wished to counter a prevalent but speculative idea that held clots to be products of inflammation. They were more likely, thought Virchow, to cause inflammation by impeding the blood flow. He was right, of course, and could demonstrate as much in experimental animals. But the theory that inflammation preceded clot formation would persist. Autopsies of patients with heart disease did not invariably yield clots in the coronary arteries, so some wondered if they mattered at all. And in the 1970s, as heart attack hit epidemic proportions, the old theory of inflammation made a remarkable comeback.

A highly influential NIH physician, William C. Roberts, prominently put forward the idea that blood clots played only a minor role—or none at all—in heart attack. Rather, he suggested, first came death of heart tissue. He suggested that "thrombi may be *consequences* rather than *causes* of [acute myocardial infarction; emphasis in original]." This interpretation became widely discussed and dampened enthusiasm for thrombolytic therapy for the best part of a decade. Heart attack, many physicians imagined, might be due to something like a coronary spasm or a damaged heart's erratic demand for blood. A clot-buster would be of no use.

But soon enough experiments demolished the theory that Roberts championed, and what happened nicely mirrored the mid-1800s, when Rudolph Virchow recovered clots after injecting them in experimental dogs. In 1980 Marcus DeWood, an internist in Spokane, Washington, published results from a series of heart attack patients whom he had subjected to coronary imaging within 24 hours after their symptoms began. He used angiography, in which a contrast agent is injected directly into the coronary arteries, followed by X-ray.

Doctors had avoided this procedure during heart attack, considering it potentially dangerous. But DeWood performed it without incident and he discovered coronary blockage in 110 of 126 patients. He could actually retrieve clots in about half that number. Still more revealing, patients who were treated later—from 12 to 24 hours after symptoms began—showed significantly less evidence of occluded arteries. The implication was clear: not only did clots cause heart attack, but the body's own fibrinolytic system worked to eliminate them. DeWood's results were rapidly replicated in a variety of venues.

Clot-busting for heart attack, in 1980, was suddenly back in vogue. Streptokinase returned to the fray, with a new protocol for administering it out of Germany. And there was renewed interest in urokinase. But by the early 1980s, another substance rapidly gained attention, due to a combination of careful science from Europe and the advent of biotech in the United States. This was the human body's endogenous clot-dissolver—liberated from tissue, purified, cloned, and produced in relative abundance. This was tPA.

Intractable all these years—from 1947, when it was discovered in slices of mammalian tissue—in 1979 tPA was isolated and purified in short order. These events both coincided with renewed interest in clot-dissolving therapy and the birth of biotech, as researchers sought to develop new drugs. Within a few months, from mid-1979 to early 1980, tPA became both potentially valuable and viable as a thrombolytic drug.

Although serendipity played a role, as Désiré Collen liked to emphasize, key too was his own intellect and collegial personality. Collen became widely identified with tPA's historic parturition. Considered brilliant and original, competitive but also highly collaborative, he was trained both as a biochemist and physician. He ran a multidisciplinary laboratory and forged close relationships with researchers in many fields, both in Europe and the United States. Many biochemists remain narrowly focused their whole careers but a few nurture larger vistas, and this surely makes sense. Individual enzymes play diverse roles in physiology, metabolism, and various diseases; there is latitude to roam.

Collen's manifold interests stemming from fibrinolytics included cancer. In 1974 he was one of several researchers to discover a molecule that prevents clots from dissolving. The presence in the blood of *alpha-2 antiplasmin*, as it was called, would rapidly—in as little as one tenth of a second—neutralize clot-dissolving plasmin. This was a contribution to basic hematology and fibrinolytics, of course, but it also held potential implications for oncology research. Various experiments with malignant tissue suggested that alpha-2 antiplasmin might hold promise as a strategy to stop tumors from growing.

"We hypothesized—it seems naive in retrospect—that antiplasmin might serve as a model," said Collen, "to develop inhibitors for malignant growth."

That was the state of affairs at the end of 1978 when a friendly visit by an American colleague to Collen's laboratory in Belgium led directly to tPA's late-blooming debut as a stand-alone molecule.

"We talked about many things," recalled Daniel B. Rifkin, a cell biologist then at Rockefeller University who, while on vacation to visit in-laws in the Netherlands, stopped by the University of Leuven to meet with Collen.

Rifkin's work involved tumor development. His recent research had shown that when normal cells turned cancerous they produced enzymatic substances—known in this context as proteases—that acted not unlike plasminogen activators. Using such a substance to digest the surrounding tissue matrix, malignant cells might reach the bloodstream and spread to distant sites—a means, in other words, for tumors to metastasize.

So among other bright topics of conversation between Rifkin and Collen that afternoon was the basic biochemistry of cancer. In particular, Collen wondered if Rifkin might know of some enzyme that would help him in further experiments with alpha-2 antiplasmin. As it happened, Rifkin said, he had recently come into possession of a cell line that exuded rather large amounts of an unusual protease. The Bowes melanoma cell line, as it was called, was named after the New York patient from whose aggressive tumor it had originally been harvested—and it would go on to join the ranks of dozens of "immortalized" cancer cells kept alive indefinitely and cultivated for research purposes and drug development. The substance the tumor produced was not urokinase, Rifkin said, which various tumors produced. But he had not investigated further.

So at the end of their visit Collen and Rifkin exchanged not only conversation but also substances. "I gave him some antiplasmin, and he gave me the Bowes melanoma cell line," recalled Collen. "*Quid pro quo*, so to speak."

The actual work on tPA thus began unwittingly. To work with the substance that the Bowes cell line produced, Collen hoped to extract and purify it. But it stubbornly remained bound within the "conditioned medium"—the exudate from the cell line. Collen tried any number of techniques. He could not extract it by freeze-drying, dialysis, or anything else. "I just couldn't purify it," he recalls, "it stuck to everything." But it was clearly present. It behaved like a plasminogen activator. To laboratory plates that contained both a fibrin clot and the cell line, adding plasminogen caused the clot to dissolve; but this was not the case in plates without plasminogen. Yet the agent that activated the plasminogen—converted it to plasmin—would not be extracted pure.

Finally, on February 13, 1979—he still remembers the day—Collen performed a simple experiment. In test tubes he combined fibrin and fibrinogen to form clots. Then to one test tube he added the exudate produced by the Bowes cell line; to another, he added urokinase. He spun the contents of each tube separately in a centrifuge. The result was a concentrated clot substance and a clear liquid, known as the supernatant—from which, Collen found, he could recover urokinase. But not a trace of the Bowes cell exudate, by contrast, could be found in the liquid. It was instead embedded in the clot. Affinity for fibrin was its salient property.

The proverbial caricature now applies: a light bulb flashed in Collen's head. He recalled: "I said, 'Bingo, this must be tPA.'" Had plasminogen been present, the clot would have dissolved. Further experiments would confirm as much. "We realized we had a cell line that everyone had been looking for."

Dan Rifkin recalls Collen's discovery with admiration and something like regret that it did not happen in his own laboratory. "The rest is history," he concluded. At the time the literature on tPA was small. "We knew that some of the properties of the melanoma plasminogen activator did not seem to be the same as the activator we got from some other tumors." Rifkin had planned for purification and had produced liters of the cell line, but the postdoctoral fellow in his lab never got around to it.

Producing pure tPA and more of it now became a high priority. Collen's research appears to have turned on a dime. As it happened, in October 1979 there arrived in his laboratory Dingeman ("Dick") Rijken, a biochemist who had previously worked with tPA. He had even managed to recover a minuscule amount of it from uterine tissue. The trick to purification turned out to be a simple detergent, widely known to chemists as Tween 80. Applied to the Bowes extract, it worked like a charm. Within a month, Collen and Rijken could say with confidence that the substance—they were still calling it melanoma plasminogen activator—was homogenous and it could not be distinguished, by any known assay, from tPA.

Collen now scaled up production, but it could never be enough. Over the next couple of years his laboratory would produce a bit more than half a teaspoonful, enough for substantive research and even a few clinical applications. Collen and colleagues both at Leuven and in the United States used it to establish that tPA could dissolve pulmonary emboli in rabbits and treat coronary artery thrombosis in experimental dogs. Humans came next—and the first among them was Willem Weimar's kidney transplant patient.

Collen sketched a larger picture, too. He suggested why tPA would more efficiently dissolve intravascular clots than either urokinase or streptokinase: it acted upon plasminogen with specificity and only in the presence of fibrin. In ordinary circulation of the blood both tPA and plasmin are inactive due to the presence of inhibitors such as alpha-2 antiplasmin. But when fibrin clots form for whatever reason, tPA binds rapidly to fibrin and converts plasminogen into clot-dissolving plasmin. By contrast, both urokinase and streptokinase were less fibrin-specific and more likely to cause bleeding. Thus, thromboembolic clots contain within themselves—as might be expected—the potential for their own ultimate dissolution.

These insights, noted Collen, had "important consequences for the development of thrombolytic agents." There now emerged the serious prospect of using tPA as a drug. Although two grams represented a thousand times more than had been produced in earlier experiments over the course of more than three decades, it was obviously insignificant in pharmaceutical terms. The Bowes cell line itself was an unlikely source. "[L]arge-scale preparation....would be at best overwhelmingly demanding and at worst, totally impractical," wrote Collen. There was, however, another solution.

Enter biotech. An alliance of biochemistry and molecular engineering, the industry we today call biotech is based on success at compelling living systems—first bacteria, later cells of more complex organisms—to manufacture pure biological products in quantity. Biotech is in effect a sophisticated advance on old-fashioned biotechnology, the more general process that includes such ancient crafts as wine- and bread-making. Indeed, in biotech one sees how humankind's furthest technological past is not really past at all; it is very near. Ancient Sumerians brewed beer and the Chinese harvested mold to salve wounds. Contemporary humans manipulate seed pods for higher crop yields and create new medicines from the stuff of DNA.

Within a few years of the first start-ups in the mid-1970s, biotech firms began to develop new drugs. From the beginning, companies with pharmaceutical aims were capital-intensive. Their business models forged links among scientists, universities, research institutions, and the larger drug companies. The complex mix of fundamental and applied research signaled an expensive proposition. Start-up companies scavenged basic research for pharmaceutical possibilities, with enzymes—such as tPA—as major targets.

In 1979, when Désiré Collen purified tPA, an early biotech avatar was the small but intellectually weighty company Genentech. One of its founders was Herb Boyer, the biochemist who in 1973, together with fellow researcher Stanley Cohen, first demonstrated what became known as recombinant genetic engineering. In Boyer and Cohen's instantly famous experiment, they created molecular clones of specific genes—that is, multiple copies of specific DNA sequences. These they extracted from the toad *Xenopus laevis* and integrated into *E. coli* bacteria. The simple deduction was that this process could compel bacteria, which divide in minutes and multiply exponentially, to fabricate ample amounts of peptides and proteins as the basis for useful drugs. Whereas most drugs were small and relatively simple molecules—aspirin is a good example—the techniques of molecular biology would now make it possible to produce complex proteins made up of strings of simpler peptides and other substances. It represented a revolutionary departure in drug design.

Persuaded by the head of research management at Stanford University, in 1974 Boyer and Cohen filed for a patent, which was eventually granted. Meanwhile, after Boyer and entrepreneur Robert Swanson created a partnership, Genentech was born in San Francisco in 1976.

Many early biotech firms failed, but Genentech was a prominent exception. In 1977 the company produced the first synthetic human protein, somatostatin, and 2 years later managed to clone it, but clinical applications would come only later. Genentech scientists also won a scientific race to clone the human gene for insulin, used to treat diabetes. Synthetic human insulin would eventually largely supplant insulin harvested from the organs of cows, to which some patients could develop allergies. Business advanced apace, and in 1980 Genentech aroused much interest on Wall Street, when its stock price leapt from $35 to $88 the day of its initial public offering—inciting visions of a new Eldorado. Genentech not coincidentally developed an aggressive legal strategy to patent and protect every single one of its molecular products; within 20 years it held more than 7,500 patents, granted or pending.

That tPA would be a candidate for Genentech's portfolio was not surprising. Like both insulin and somatostatin, it was the product of a single—albeit large—gene. Like them, too, it was a natural substance of a specific type common to mammals. However, where recombinant insulin would simply replace an animal analogue and somatostatin would be used to treat a relatively uncommon condition, tPA was poised to be a genuinely novel drug for major disorders. With heart attack at epidemic proportions—an average of one every 20 seconds, 588 deaths per 100,000 annually in the United States in 1980—and renewed responsibility laid to thrombi and emboli in the vast majority of cases, recombinant tPA could be a breakthrough. And, although nobody was yet thinking much about it, the same was true for stroke.

Genentech's actual decision to find out more about tPA was due to Herb Heynecker, a Dutch biochemist, one of the original Genentech scientists and later a businessman. Reading the literature on urokinase, which Genentech had contracted to clone just because tiny purified amounts of it already existed, he happened upon tPA. Now, he learned, it too was said to have been extracted and purified. Heynecker immediately recognized the potential and told colleagues that it "sounds even more interesting than urokinase."

Thus, within just a few months after shedding its reputation as a thoroughly elusive enzyme, tPA was suddenly of interest to the rising field of biotech.

The fast pace of the tPA story from this point onward indicates a culture shift as prospects for exploiting a single protein molecule left the exclusively academic domain and entered a research atmosphere funded by venture capital. The drive to develop tPA as a drug would be costly, labor-intensive, and precipitated by competition. The "curiosity-driven" model then common in university-based medical research would be supplanted—for better or worse, or both—by one that valued results and marketability.

The science at Genentech—some would say, as opposed to the rapacious marketing—was always excellent. When Herb Heynecker moved to find out more about tPA in June 1980, he dispatched Diane Pennica, a newly hired young PhD, to a European congress on fibrinolysis, held in the wake of the Collen laboratory's newly minted discoveries. Pennica arrived early in Malmo, Sweden, introduced herself to Collen, and explained why she was there. The charismatic, ever-sociable scientist invited her to join him and other investigators to dinner. On the spot, inasmuch as the mammalian gene that produced tPA had been identified, Pennica brashly suggested that Genentech would clone it. Once cloned, it could be churned out in quantity and tested as a possible clot-busting drug.

Collen was skeptical, pointing out that the tPA gene was quite large. (The gene for insulin, for example, was relatively small, with 51 amino acids; that for tPA was ten times as big.) Yet Pennica was as insistent and convincing as she was young and attractive—she looked about 17 years old, colleagues recalled, while conveying intelligence and competence. In the end Collen agreed. He would provide the purified tPA/melanoma protein under a contractual agreement.

"I didn't tell him that I had never cloned anything in my life," recalls Pennica.

Today, cloning a gene of 2,530 base pairs of DNA for a protein that consists of 527 amino acids would be largely automated and take a few days at most. Not so in 1980. The process was one of painstaking reverse engineering. The long chain of amino acids that makes up the protein had to be deconstructed and back-translated into the genetic code embedded in the nucleotide sequences of DNA. The unique gene itself had to be sought within the genome, sequenced in its entirety, and then shown to work as promised. Details of Pennica's work are beyond the scope of this book, but after 6 months of intensive work her laboratory produced a single, incomplete match between a short DNA sequence and a series of amino acids in a fragment of tPA. Another half-year's work and the full sequence was worked out. Pennica and her group confirmed that the human genome contains a single gene that codes for tPA, provided its complete sequence and structure, and demonstrated it performed as promised. She would present the results at the sixth International Congress on Fibrinolysis in

Lausanne, Switzerland, in July 1982, and her paper was published in *Nature* the following January.

The way now opened to the development of recombinant tPA (r-tPA). A molecule that had worked silently and anonymously for millions of years as part of a system that dissolves blood clots in mammalian circulation now entered a new phase in its natural history. Together with advances in medicine that clarified the physiology of heart attack and stroke, tPA was poised to become a powerful drug.

Dead or Alive | 3

*J*ustin A. Zivin, in early 1984, received a flat turndown. Only experiment could decide if tPA might be good to treat stroke. So could Genentech spare a few vials? A brief phone conversation brought a pointed response. Elliott Grossbard, board certified in both internal medicine and hematology, also held a law degree from Yale. He was the Genentech executive charged with shepherding the drug through clinical trials for heart attack. Not stroke.

"I trained with Raymond Adams at Massachusetts General Hospital," he told Zivin curtly, mentioning one of the most prominent neurologists of the mid-20th century. "He taught us that stroke is not treatable."

Even if Zivin had been a senior scientist or a known quantity to Genentech, the answer would probably have been the same. As it happened, he was relatively junior, with some experience at the National Institutes of Health but unknown to drug discovery. In any event his interest in performing animal experiments with tPA—"He wanted to do a clot in a rabbit," remembers Grossbard dismissively—was not in accord with the company's agenda. Trials with heart attack patients were just getting under way. Hope for success ran high; so too did fear of failure: "We were concerned he would do the experiment, report intracerebral hemorrhage subsequent to dissolving the clot, and we'd end up with a safety issue."

Zivin held appointments as associate professor in the departments of neurology and pharmacology at the University of Massachusetts. At 37 he was both a research physiologist and clinical neurologist. The first he heard of tPA came by a mundane source: his Sunday newspaper. It merited a brief discussion in a lengthy article about scientific and business prospects for the new biotech companies. "The Selling of Science" appeared in the *Boston Globe* in late August 1983, the cover story in the newspaper's magazine. "Biotechnology is more than designer genes," advised the callout. "It's a high-stakes business with competitors and a bottom line."

Not current with biotech, what Zivin knew of molecular biology was limited to the essentials taught in medical school. In years since he had heard about the promise of bioengineered molecules. His own research, which had recently begun to stray from the strictly biochemical side of neurology, was distinguished by its statistical slant. Only vaguely was he aware of the frenzy to develop everything from improved rennet for cheese to vaccines for pigs. He knew that biotech was bruited to be the holy grail of drug discovery, but the way he read matters, so far as the brain was concerned, not a great deal was yet useful to know. That view, in late summer 1983, proved due for revision.

"There are times," wrote Monty Montgomery in the *Globe*, "when doctors would like to be able to dissolve [clots] quickly—during heart attacks, during blood-clotting crises in the brain (strokes), when painful clots strike the veins of the legs, or when life-threatening blood clots reach the lungs."

The phrase *blood-clotting crises in the brain* naturally gained Zivin's attention, as did clot-dissolving enzymes found in human tissue—known as plasminogen activators. Urokinase—found years before in urine, hence the name—was under investigation by Victor Guervich at Tufts University School of Medicine. The other, tPA, was being manufactured by the South San Francisco-based company Genentech, with perhaps some competitors in the background. The promise of a drug that offered "the first practical way to dissolve blood clots in now inaccessible arteries to the brain" was an arresting idea that Zivin did not know how to evaluate.

But "The Selling of Science" was only a tantalizing newspaper story and as much about business as drug discovery. After reading it, Zivin talked with Marc Fisher, a neurologist more familiar than he was with hematology and in closer touch with research cardiologists. Fisher knew that for tPA in particular the target was heart attack and right there on campus, at the University of Massachusetts Medical School, cardiologist Joel Gore was a principal investigator in a large controlled study. Some patients would receive tPA while others would get the older drug, streptokinase. Known as Thrombolysis in Myocardial Infarction (TIMI), the study was just getting under way.

There matters rested so far as Zivin was concerned—a few shreds of information about a new clot-busting substance—for several months. But the message transmitted by the *Globe* story was not lost: a new substance, an endogenous human enzyme, held potential as a treatment for heart attack. There was no doubt it ought to be of interest as well for acute stroke.

In 1984 Zivin was primed for a shift in focus. At the university he had a small animal laboratory in the basement of the building where he worked and, upstairs, a biochemical lab across from his office. Like everyone in neurology, he was aware of the lack of progress in stroke treatments and felt the press of frustration. Not long before, after presenting some arcane information on spinal cord ischemia at a pharmacology seminar, his friend and mentor Doug Waud had chided him afterward.

"Those were data," said Waud, "that only a mother could love."

The jibe was meant as a joke, but Zivin did not take it that way. He was hurt and angry. But in time he acknowledged Waud was right: the research he had presented was indeed of little use to anybody. From the beginning of his career he wanted to work with clinical possibilities. He had shifted away from spinal cord trauma after realizing that future advances in that field would come from neurosurgeons. He turned to stroke but now recognized he had become bogged down in biochemical esoterica.

Training as a scientist and physician had meant for Zivin a blend of dependence on personal heritage and a desire to be separate and independent of it. His father Simon was an internist and his uncle—his father's identical twin, Israel—was a neurologist. In Chicago he had grown up bored when he accompanied his father on house calls. But he was intrigued when, clad in green scrubs, he observed surgeries; he was nauseated but determined while watching autopsies. He nurtured an identity in science. An early interest in astronomy ended only when he discovered he was more attuned to biology than to physics. So he went to medical school after all, but without sacrificing his allegiance to science and the laboratory. He emerged from the Medical Scientist Training Program at Northwestern University with both a medical degree and a PhD in physiology.

Zivin had grown up in Chicago during the 1950s, when a bright child might well combine a durable set of insecurities with a measure of intellectual arrogance. "That somber city," as Saul Bellow called it, marked for life its natives because insignificance was everyone's presumed destiny; overcoming it required insolence. Unlike New York or San Francisco, Midwestern cities confined intellect to the university campus; they were too filled with industry and commerce. "Physically, it was a monochromatic gray," wrote Alan Erenhalt of Chicago in *The Lost City*. After World War II, the colorful immigrant generations were fading away. "Residents and newcomers alike made conversation in the 1950s about Chicago's overpowering drabness." A Second City childhood did not necessarily make intelligent men comfortable in the wider world. Zivin was no exception: insecurities, he later said, affected him well into his forties.

But there was always a counterbalance of gall. The clinical literature on stroke, Zivin thought, was defective. The lack of rigor was self-evident to anyone who paged through the journals. Still in vogue was the case-study approach, in which authors would typically discuss perplexing patients in clever ways to no useful end. If others had misgivings, Zivin was something of a cheerless bomb-thrower. As a resident at the University of California, San Francisco, he once voiced his global view to his department chair. Asked why he didn't cite the literature in writing or teaching, he replied that it was lousy. He read it, but it was fundamentally defective. In a world with an ever-more-solid grasp of biochemical dynamics, clinical neurology stuck itself with a limited descriptive model that was basically phenomenological, not scientific. That was not good enough.

"But it's all we've got," replied the chairman.

After receiving his doctorates in 1971 and 1972, Zivin worked at the National Institute of Mental Health to fulfill military service as the war in Vietnam wound down. He went to San Francisco for his residency before moving with his wife and two children, in 1978, to the University of Massachusetts. His department chairman, neurologist David Drachman, remembered he was eager to begin research when he arrived, and shortly thereafter he started work on the first of his rabbit models for stroke: "He probably set up his laboratory here faster than anybody else I've ever recruited."

In late autumn 1984, several months after "The Selling of Science" appeared in the *Boston Globe*, Zivin learned of an event that might answer some of his questions about tPA. At nearby Harvard University an *ad hoc* group calling itself the Thrombolysis Forum of Greater Boston announced a meeting set for December 5, 1983. The public was invited, with speakers to include two scientists unknown to him: Désiré Collen, apparently an international star in fibrinolytics research, and Diane Pennica, a young scientist at Genentech. They would discuss plasminogen activators and recombinant DNA technology.

From the wooden title, "Thrombolysis: Whither Goes the Field?" one might not realize that the tPA bandwagon was coming to town—the early trumpetings of a potentially high-power drug from biotech. But so it was. Zivin and Marc Fisher decided to attend.

A common disease without an effective treatment that gives rise to a climate of negative opinion is sometimes called "therapeutic nihilism"—when doctors cannot do anything useful. While discoveries in such fields as physiology add knowledge, they only increase frustration. Nothing beneficial could be done for a stroke victim in 1983. But Elliott Grossbard's view that stroke was untreatable was both factual and a reflection of excessively low expectations.

In fact, several recent advances pointed away from gloomy and tenacious therapeutic nihilism. A stroke had come to be understood as a "brain attack" on a par with, and often closely related to, heart attack. The ratio of ischemic (occlusive) to hemorrhagic (bleeding) strokes was now known to be about eight to one, perhaps more. In addition, imaging the brain and cerebral vasculature had become simpler in the late 1970s, after the advent of computerized tomography (CT). Because CT scans could reliably and immediately detect cerebral hemorrhage, they could also, by deduction and in conjunction with symptom evaluation, furnish fast diagnosis of ischemic stroke.

It was true, though, that positive news was thus far confined to prevention. Death from stroke had declined over the course of 30 years or more, plainly due to drug therapy to treat high blood pressure, now understood as a potent risk factor. Aspirin might play a useful role in avoiding strokes because it was understood to inhibit the way that cell fragments known as platelets contributed to clot formation and clogging or hardening of the arteries. Studies were under way to test whether aspirin ought to be prescribed after a transient ischemic attack (TIA)—the mild event after which patients seemed to be at greater risk for a serious stroke. Similarly, vasodilators—drugs that relaxed and widened blood vessels—were also being studied with a view to prevention.

Yet the simple fact remained that stroke, the third most common killer after heart attack and all forms of cancer combined, was the leading cause of neurological disability. For acute ischemic stroke—the event as it happened—the picture remained stark and grim. "No specific drug treatment for cerebral infarction is of proven value," wrote Vladimir Hachinski and John W. Norris in *The Acute Stroke*, a book published in 1985, "and many time-hallowed methods are useless or harmful and should be abandoned." Efforts to reduce pressure inside the cranium had been tried and found useless. Trials with barbiturates, steroids, and vasoconstrictive drugs had come up negative.

Physicians did still employ anticoagulant drugs to treat stroke. Why? Patients were frequently prescribed heparin—they were "heparinized"—in spite of growing evidence it did not work. Anticoagulants reduced circulating fibrin but could do nothing to dissolve thrombi or emboli already formed. All the randomized studies were negative. One conclusion can stand for all: "[F]rom the standpoint of mortality, anticoagulant therapy plays no beneficial role in the treatment of thrombotic cerebrovascular disease and may be harmful." Nevertheless, hope persisted and in retrospect surpassed reason; the fact these drugs were long promoted by leading lights in neurology perhaps proved too compelling. Prescribing anticoagulants after a stroke in the 1980s represented a late example of what the famous physician William Osler called "popgun pharmacy"—using a drug without knowing if it works. Trials of heparin and other anticoagulants would continue into the 21st century.

"Thrombolysis: Whither Goes the Field?" was just one of many events at which Désiré Collen presented his research and work in developing tPA. By 1983 he had furthered his initial success. In addition to treating kidney transplant patients, collaborations in Belgium and the United States brought more promising results. Numbers were small—six of seven patients had their occluded arteries opened with tPA—but this work proved the concept and now large multicenter heart trials were starting. Development of tPA would become Collen's major scientific achievement in clinical medicine.

Diane Pennica, from Genentech, also spoke at the forum. Facing the crowded auditorium, she might have recalled the meeting in Lausanne, Switzerland, in June 1982 when she reported sequencing the tPA gene. Before she attended that event, Genentech had pledged her to secrecy. The abstract for her paper concealed more than it revealed. Her presentation had been scheduled for the tail end of the meeting and coincided with the moment the company issued a press release. Now, by stark contrast, she was talking to overflow audiences in a mood of growing excitement. A bandwagon of opinion was taking on passengers; anticipation was growing.

Zivin would later recall the atmosphere pervading the packed Sherman Auditorium at Beth Israel Hospital. Although stroke was not on the agenda, this was the event that viscerally energized him. Until then he had been only vaguely aware that fibrinolytic agents such as streptokinase—about which he knew almost nothing—were contraindicated for stroke. Heparin he understood did not work. But a recombinant drug that cloned the body's own clot-dissolving enzyme was perhaps something quite different.

Where were the neurologists? With all the disappointment around stroke?

A few weeks later he had telephoned Genentech, and Elliot Grossbard rebuffed his request for tPA. Genentech left the door cracked open, however. After Grossbard's categorical negative, Zivin, persistent, wrote him a letter the same day. He attached a proposal suggesting how tPA for "appropriate types of stroke" might be tested. Three weeks later came a reply from the preclinical studies coordinator: "Although interesting," B. J. Marafino wrote, his plan for animal studies did not "constitute an area of investigation that Genentech intends to explore in the near future." But, he added, the drug might be forthcoming in 6 to 9 months "[a]s product development progresses."

Although Zivin was not aware of it at the time, there was more to the story. Together with a research hematologist, Laurence Harker, Désiré Collen had visited Genentech and suggested treating individual stroke patients in an experimental setting, just as had been done at first with heart attack.

"I thought that at the moment it was somewhat too high a risk for the program," recalled Grossbard. Because streptokinase for heart attack elevated the risk of cerebral hemorrhage, the same might be true of tPA. Again, such a failure could derail or retard FDA approval. So Grossbard said no, and Harker backed off.

In retrospect, decision-makers at Genentech from the start were both drawn to the concept of tPA for stroke but apprehensive about any possible interference with its use in myocardial infarction, the disorder expected to constitute its most lucrative market if and when it was green-lighted. They were also aware of lurking competition from other companies. In months and years to come, Genentech would repeatedly evince ambivalence around tPA for stroke. Saying no to Zivin had meant "not now"; it did not mean never.

Absence of a treatment for stroke was all the more aggravating because basic research had not neglected the brain. In fact, scientists worked with an ever-deeper understanding of it, in sickness and in health, via molecular biology and biochemistry. An increasingly sophisticated description of brain metabolism had emerged during the 1960s and 1970s, together with an account of the chemical mishaps that occur during ischemic stroke, often with lethal consequences. No one in 1983 knew it all—details are still being sought today—but advances were substantial.

The key series of events during a stroke, today commonly called the "ischemic cascade," begins when cerebral circulation is suddenly reduced in some part of the brain. As blood-deprived tissue rapidly exhausts available oxygen and glucose, cell membranes begin to fall apart. Calcium ions that are normally embedded within two cellular structures, the mitochondria and endoplasmic reticulum, flow willy-nilly throughout nerve cells. There they remain in massive amounts. "The well-contained fire in the hearth thus spreads to involve the entire house," wrote William K. Hass in a classic account. Damage that free calcium provokes in nerve tissue, first noted in the early 20th century, had come under intensive study. What once was called "softening of the brain"—the term an index of perplexity—was now termed "infarct" and known to arise from chemical changes more or less well understood.

Importantly, this new knowledge pointed to a time factor. For years scientists had believed, and doctors learned, that in just minutes damage to brain tissue from ischemia could be irreversible. Recent research challenged this view while, unlike previous advances, detailed biochemistry actually pointed to new and unprecedented prospects for treatment. Damage, it seemed, might in many instances be undone and avoided. Although dead tissue could not be returned to life, the ischemic cascade was understood to take place over several hours; damage need not be measured in seconds.

A time window, real if not large, was generally acknowledged by clinicians in 1983, and Zivin put numbers to it. In 1982 he put forward a novel method he used to mimic ischemic stroke in humans. In a rabbit he installed a "snare ligature" around the abdominal aorta—the largest of the arteries from the heart—so that the experimenter, simply by tugging on a string, could cut off circulation to the nervous system. Such controlled obstruction of blood flow simulated ischemic stroke. Whether an animal recovered or was subject to permanent paralysis, Zivin was able to show, strongly correlated with how long circulation was impeded. He showed too that deficits might be reversible. On this view, the mild transient ischemic attack (TIA) would not be a separate disease but, rather, on a continuum with the more serious stroke-in-evolution. Although people walked away from TIAs while serious strokes resulted in disability or death, the events at bottom were the same. All this meant, he noted, new prospects for "pharmacological strategies" that could minimize "the damage caused by [central nervous system] ischemia."

And for acute stroke, tPA might provide just such a strategy. Had its potential been less promising, Zivin might have moved on to something else. Certainly, without cooperation from Genentech, "I was stuck," he observed years later. But he decided to go forward with plans to create a new animal model to test tPA even though he had no certainty of obtaining it.

The task occupied him for a year. His rabbit model for spinal cord ischemia only mimicked stroke. Zivin now required more than a simulation. He would inject genuine clots inside the cerebral vasculature to create strokes and see whether tPA made them better. For statistical evaluation, the clots themselves must be of known size and weight. Such a model, and a system for inducing stroke in a controlled fashion, did not exist.

Indeed, the animal models popular in stroke research in 1983 constituted yet another index of the lack of rigor in the field. Dozens of different models all tried to do the same thing: mimic some type of human stroke with the aim of establishing morphological endpoints—that is, associate dead brain tissue in specific locations with behavioral deficits. Researchers might induce stroke in some part of the brain—often, a rat's—by cutting off circulation in some artery, then outline the lesion and measure the damage. Other models attempted to catalogue behavioral deficits without any effort at quantitative measurement at all. The experiments were cumbersome, labor-intensive, and not very informative; those using actual clots were notoriously ineffective. Predicting where a small clot was going to lodge in a monkey's brain, for example, was impossible. With a larger clot, one might be right about where it would go, but not about how much damage it would cause: a hefty clot landing in a capacious vessel might not cause an infarct at all.

Finally and above all, none of the common models had any implications for treatment; they were academic, often redundant exercises. To learn how a hole in an animal's brain affected its behavior opened no road to therapy; it bore minimal hope of helping any human being afflicted by stroke.

In setting out to build a better model and to design experiments with tPA, Zivin employed a statistical method that, although not new, was novel to neurology. He had used it with his spinal cord experiments, but it was otherwise unknown in stroke research. *Quantal dose-response analysis*, as the method was called, would add rigor and efficiency to animal experiments. Its essence was to avoid unnecessary complexity by asking simple questions and obtaining robust answers.

In science, complicated problems burdened with many unknowns require, especially at the outset, a simplifying approach. In the 1840s Rudolph Virchow, in connection with his own pioneering research on intravascular blood clots, which could not be located except at autopsy, had noted as much. With a deficient body of knowledge, he wrote, if "one asks detailed questions one receives, often enough, a Delphic answer only." Something similar was going on in neurology some 140 years later, with useless efforts to generalize from the tangled web of events that occur in any particular stroke. In contrast, Zivin developed experiments in which a small number of animals could supply a great deal of information about many, many strokes.

He had come to this juncture by an unexpected insight into how stroke might be visualized. One day in 1979, looking over some pharmacological data while studying for his neurology board exams, it suddenly occurred to Zivin that "dose-response plots" for drugs could be equally well used to describe what happened with stroke. Such charts use a sigmoid curve—sometimes called an S curve—to show the efficacy of a drug from low to maximum doses. The shape of the response could also be used to visualize ischemic stroke, with its various outcomes over time ranging from no deficit to death.

Intuitively, the concept is easy to grasp: a drug will start to work beginning at some threshold dose but will eventually reach a point at which a higher dose will have no additional impact. Ischemic stroke, Zivin recognized, would follow the same pattern.

"If you made something ischemic for a short period of time, there wouldn't be any damage and we knew that. But as you start to get onto the fast-rising part of the curve, the more ischemia you have, the more damage you cause.

Ultimately you get to the top, and the curve flattens out again because there's no more possibility of doing any damage."

At the bottom of the S curve, no damage; at the top, maximal destruction and death. Although he recognized how stroke fitted the sigmoid shape, Zivin also realized that he did not know how to perform the statistical analysis that could measure it. If he could do that, he would have not only a picture of stroke but a means to test agents to treat it. Through experiments he could compare data sets; the curves for a drug that in fact worked would significantly differ from those of the control.

Analytic help came through the work and person of Doug Waud, a pharmacologist at the University of Massachusetts who became his friend, colleague, and mentor. Zivin's own interest in statistics was not new—in 1976 he had published a paper with the title "Statistics for Disinterested Scientists"—but his relationship with Waud purchased a whole new level of understanding. Eventually they wrote several articles together, one of which practically gave a short course to stroke researchers on the use of statistics.

In the wake of a stroke, human patients show tremendous variability in symptoms depending on the location, size, and character of the infarct, but the situation in animals such as rats and rabbits is much different: they evince only a few visible signs or measurable behaviors. However, this apparent drawback can actually be turned to great advantage. It favors a reductionist approach that can eliminate unnecessary information in order to more closely focus on the essential question as to whether a drug—tPA, for example—succeeds or fails in restoring blood flow. The question to ask is simple: Is the animal normal? Or is it comatose or dead? Yes or no? This non-graded but discontinuous, dead-or-alive approach made sense for experiments, of course, only if the clots could be controlled as to number, as to size, and as to dispersion within the cerebral vasculature. Zivin would not try to introduce one clot into many animals—a strategy that frequently led to no pathological effect—but to put many clots into a few animals.

In a sense, the rabbit model he finally came up with—working through the math with Waud—was the opposite of most animal stroke experiments, which essentially involved only counting (numbers of animals, size of infarcts, numbers of deficits) followed by a simple test to gauge significance. The rabbit model, by contrast, was designed to test drugs during acute stroke. Small groups of animals could be dosed with large numbers of clots that caused multiple strokes and then, from the answers to a simple question (Are you dead or alive?), could be generated a sigmoid curve.

Comparing that curve with another in which the animals were also stroked but, in addition, dosed with a therapeutic agent would reveal whether the drug was effective. Results with treated animals versus controls would yield a robust percentage based on probability. When colleagues were skeptical, as they sometimes were, Zivin finally came up with a baseball analogy. "In baseball, you get a hit or you don't. If you're successful a third of the time, you can be extraordinarily well paid. But if you're successful 20% of the time, it's time to look for a new job."

Good news came late in 1984 when Marc Fisher, after a trip to San Francisco and meeting with Elliott Grossbard, managed to obtain a small amount of tPA. Zivin could now carry out the experiments he had been planning ever since "Thrombolysis: Whither Goes the Field?" The new rabbit model to send blood clots directly into the cerebral vasculature was ready. The process was simple: anesthetize the rabbits, sew a plastic catheter into the carotid artery (the main circulatory conduit to the brain), cap it, then allow the animals to wake up. This was the clot injection system. Just two dozen rabbits were all he needed—12 for tPA, 12 for controls; each animal would receive from 2,100 to 3,600 clots.

Fabricating clots of the same size and making them uniform had proved troublesome. Zivin settled on a method by which he extracted blood from a donor animal, allowed it to coagulate, then fragmented it in a blender-like instrument known as a Polytron. Near uniform-sized clots had to be variable in weight by batch, and so he developed a system for sifting them accordingly. Mesh screens manufactured by a toy train company turned out to work fine. To calculate the numbers of clots in the solution to be injected, he adapted a device known as a hemocytometer, used for counting blood cells.

Clot clumping created a problem at first. When bathed in standard solutions for injection, the thousands of small clots would re-coagulate like mud. It turned out that this was due to electrostatic charges that made the clots act like tiny magnets. The eventual answer was to soak the clots in a solution that conferred a neutral charge on all.

The key experiments took place over 2 weeks in April 1985. On each weekday two or three pairs of rabbits would be chosen: one of each pair to receive clots plus tPA; the other, a control, to receive only clots. The same batch of clots in suspension served each pair. Zivin, blinded to the results, neither injected the animals nor administered the tPA or placebo. Lab technicians in his basement laboratory performed those tasks, and they too were blinded as to which animals received tPA or a simple saline solution. For each animal, two observers would independently grade the animals to assess neurological function. One of them would not be present when the animals were treated, and so was blinded to the injection regimen, but in any event there were no discrepancies in evaluation.

When he received the first set of data on a Friday afternoon, Zivin ran a preliminary analysis. It was strongly positive: a significant difference showed up between the tPA and control groups. As for the magnitude, though, he could not tell. He did not say anything to anybody, but that weekend was as exciting as any he had ever spent as a scientist. (He did not even tell his wife, who was angry about it later.) Not often does research yield data that could help change the way medicine works. He managed as best he could not to think about what was happening. As a medical student, he had taught himself to suppress powerful emotions; he could not otherwise tolerate dealing with hopeless cancer patients, for example, or young children tearfully pleading with him over the simplest intervention. Now he put that ability to use. But he told himself: "If this goes on next week, we're really going to have something."

Experiments in science, whether one reads about them or even witnesses them as an outside observer, can appear perplexing, bizarre, minimal. Nothing seems to happen, or not much. Seldom does an experiment bring forth a huge result obvious to all—the atomic bomb being a notable exception. Louis Pasteur, in experiments to deflate the theory that life can start by spontaneous generation, with his flair for drama, declaimed before large audiences: "And I wait, I watch, I question it, begging it to recommence for me the beautiful spectacle of the first creation."

He was talking about a flask of sterile air. Just as undramatic would have been the sight of Ernest Rutherford in 1907, watching occasional sparks fly off a piece of gold foil. Rutherford famously realized that it was "as if you had fired a fifteen-inch shell at a piece of tissue paper and it came back and hit you"—and now he knew the structure of the atom. For that matter, consider the "bingo" moment when Désiré Collen deduced that the stuff exuded by a melanoma cell line was actually tPA. That discovery depended on *not* finding something in a fluid.

Such observational dissonance owes to the fact that science is a "high context" activity. Part of the message that any experiment conveys is formulated in the external world—in the lab setup, the behavior of an animal, some clinical sign or symptom. But the more weighty and explanatory part of the message— the key to success or failure—lies within the experimenter: it is intellectual and cognitive, not visible or tactile.

One of the observers on the rabbit experiments was Joan Stashak, a biochemist who worked as a technician in Zivin's laboratory in the mid-1980s. She would rate the animals after they were stroked with clots, when they would immediately become paraplegic; she would observe them again a day later, recording each time which of the animals had reflexes and which did not. The animals were numbered and she recalled observing one in particular that seemed seriously affected: "When I saw the limpness in the reflexes of the rabbit, I mean, that animal was stroked." Returning the next day she remembers

her surprise at finding it alive and active: "I just said, 'Hey, that guy's normal.'"
She too was blinded, of course: "I didn't know which ones had tPA and which
ones didn't."

To Zivin, the experiment's power was coiled in the statistics themselves,
much as if it were an experiment in physics. Its potency seemed to multiply a
thousand-fold when he had the final results and performed the analysis at the
end of the second week.

Impressive numbers stood out. Of the 11 rabbits that had received tPA, 10
were classified as normal both at 24 hours and again when checked a week later.
But in the control group of 12 animals, 4 were dead within a day and 3 others
showed grossly abnormal features. In other words, to the single dead-or-alive
question, 10 of 11 rabbits receiving tPA answered "Yes." For the control group,
the number was 5 of 12.

Quantal dose-response analysis revealed still more striking evidence. Clots
varied in size by batch, with total weight of clots from 15 to 150 milligrams. So
many clots were injected into each rabbit that they could be expected to create
multiple strokes in any given brain. For the control animals, the average weight
of clots required to produce a serious deficit or death in half of the control animals turned out to be 45.3 milligrams. By contrast, half the tPA-treated animals
could withstand clots that weighed up to 75.7 milligrams—larger and heavier
by about 60%.

Zivin finished the experiment by analyzing brain tissue from both sets of
animals. He confirmed there were infarcts but no significant hemorrhages, and
established in test tubes that tPA actually acted to dissolve the clots. He worked
up the results into a paper that he sent off to *Science*.

By then, about September 1985, Zivin had closed his laboratories at the
University of Massachusetts and moved with his wife and children to San Diego,
where he took up new posts—as associate professor at the University of
California and a physician with the Veterans Administration Medical Center.
Soon after, *Science* editors telephoned him to say they wanted to publish "Tissue
Plasminogen Activator Reduces Neurological Damage After Stroke Embolism."
The article appeared in short order, in the issue of December 13, 1985.

The rabbit model tPA experiment represented the first step toward a novel
therapy for acute stroke. It might have won more attention at the time, but
nationally the big science-and-medicine story that week concerned some gene
therapy experiments at the NIH—which, like most such research, turned out
to be nothing later on. "Those guys," recalled Zivin, "were good at PR, and
I was not."

But whether academic neurologists would respond positively, Zivin could
only hope. He knew that, on the medical side of the ledger, his work was meeting

with resistance. Quantal analysis helped him introduce rigor into stroke research, and publication of the tPA paper in *Science* represented a vindication of that approach, but it did not translate into acceptance. Some viewed his spinal cord model as crude, and they probably thought the same thing about his research with tPA. He was aware, as he and Doug Waud put it, that "the statistical literature is frequently very technical and therefore not easily assimilated by scientists who are concerned with biological questions...."

Although it may sound strange because medical information so often is communicated to the public through numbers, doctors in the 1980s were uncomfortable with statistics. In many respects they still are today. Although told to count for more than 150 years and taught that measurements of all sorts illuminate multiple aspects of biology and genetics, doctors tend to harbor a layer of hostility. And not only them: biologists, too. Zivin remembered a talk he gave when he was a research associate at the National Institute of Mental Health in the 1970s, during which he mentioned using the "Student's t-test." In the audience was Jules Axelrod, a Nobel laureate for his work on neurotransmitters, who asked him: "Why don't you use the professional version?"

There exists no such thing. The "Student's t-test" is just the simplest way to estimate statistical confidence in small samples. It was so named by William Sealy Gosset, a chemist with the Guinness Brewery whose employer regarded the use of statistics in beer-making as a trade secret and so demanded Gosset's anonymity in his publications.

In any event, no matter how matters were viewed, the paper in *Science* constituted a clear brief in favor of human clinical trials for tPA. A couple of dozen rabbits had suggested that time was a key factor and also shown once again how stroke, in terms of simple mechanics, was not much more complicated than plumbing.

Other research tended in the same direction. Hematologists Gregory del Zoppo and Laurence Harker, together with researchers in Germany, were publishing results of experimental thrombolysis for stroke with baboons; they were soon to try urokinase and streptokinase in humans. These small uncontrolled, observational studies by themselves carried limited weight, but they were positive signposts for thrombolysis. And now that tPA was gaining considerable prominence in trials to treat heart attack, it was also becoming a logical focus for stroke. Whether it could be used to obliterate cerebral blood clots now became a question for which only a randomized, controlled study could provide the answer.

Brain-O | 4

*T*om Brott came armed with two magnums: one a fine dry Champagne and the other a bottle of the sweet wine known best to binge-drinking alcoholics as Mad Dog 20-20. He brought them both to the Airlie Conference Center in Warrenton, Virginia, one weekend in August 1995, when three dozen researchers gathered to learn the results of their long-awaited study to evaluate tPA for stroke. There was apprehension: stroke trials had disappointed so often that a new study could not bear the weight of much hope. Champagne would be popped if the trials were positive, Mad Dog slugged in dismay if results were negative.

Bucolic surroundings may also have leavened the tone. The Airlie Conference Center—billed as an "island of thought"—was isolated from nearby Washington, D.C. Deer and wild geese roamed its 250 acres, landscaped to create an atmosphere conducive to cooperation and reflection. A new butterfly garden housed the Tiger Swallowtail, the Cabbage White, and Great Spangled Fritillary. Nevertheless, the place struck one of the younger neurologists as more like a CIA safe house—sparely furnished bedrooms, neither televisions nor telephones. The data were sequestered in a locked room, with a fellow posted outside.

John Marler, project director for the NINDS stroke study, belittled any notion of high security. He had chosen Airlie simply because it was a nice place and, whatever the outcome, the group would work collectively on an article based on the results.

41

Yet it was also true that Genentech executives had expressed a desire to trumpet a press release immediately after the results were revealed, should they prove positive. Such publicity was not to be. Study leaders explained to Juergen Froehlich, the company representative, that Genentech must wait for publication of the results in the prestigious *New England Journal of Medicine*. Success, it was hoped, would provoke swift action by the FDA. Although tPA was already approved for heart attack, a significant change in labeling would be required before Genentech could advertise it for acute stroke.

Most people arrived the night before the results were to be exposed. In addition to John Marler came his boss, Michael Walker, who ran the stroke division at the National Institute of Neurological Disorders and Stroke (NINDS). So, too, the local principal investigators from eight medical centers across the country. Members of the Data Safety and Monitoring Committee were present, together with K. M. A.("Mike") Welch, the clinician who ran the study's Coordinating Center at Henry Ford Health Sciences Center in Detroit.

After breakfast, recalled Patrick Lyden, the local principal investigator from the University of California San Diego, "We all assembled in the room and you practically could hear a drum roll."

Chief statistician and the Coordinating Center's principal investigator, Barbara Tilley, and her assistant, Mei Lu, were alone in knowing results of the extensive statistical workup. Even study administrators were not privy to the final numbers. Neurologists who had blindly treated stroke patients for 4 years with either tPA or a placebo could only suspect. Some later said they had intimations; others disdained any appeal to intuition.

At the head of the room Tom Brott displayed the bottles of Champagne and wine and turned to Tilley. Which should he open?

"Well, we did it," she said.

She flashed the basic numbers on an overhead projector.

A dropped-jaw moment when no one knew what to say.

Tilley added: "Open the Champagne."

Today, more than a dozen years on, the NINDS Stroke Study remains the first successful, robust, and most frequently cited of all efforts to test tPA for ischemic stroke. Researchers continue to mine the original data. The study consisted of two trials—randomized, controlled, and double-blind. Subjects were stroke victims who were treated (or not) and followed over time. The size was moderate, in terms of the number of patients, but the treatment effect was large and highly significant. For all the consternation to follow, Barbara Tilley exposed numbers to neurologists at Airlie that represented a powerfully positive outcome such as had never been seen in stroke therapy.

"It was a remarkable moment," said Mike Welch, "the first time ever that anything had ever proven to be effective for acute stroke."

For almost 4 years, from early 1991 through early 1995, at eight university medical centers and some 40 hospitals around the country, NINDS researchers treated strokes as acute emergencies. On call around the clock, doctors sped to treat with no idea whether they were giving tPA or doing nothing for individual patients. They knew only that the data they submitted were monitored, so if they were causing significant harm, the study would be stopped. Aided by nurses, radiologists, and emergency personnel, they evaluated urgent cases and administered either tPA or a placebo within either of two remarkably short time frames of 90 and 180 minutes after symptom onset. For every patient who qualified and consented, they would see and evaluate many more who had to be excluded. For the field of stroke neurology in the United States, the trial represented an unprecedented collective expenditure of time and effort.

But the NINDS study was not pure success—and therein lies its compelling interest. Publication of the paper that analyzed its results in the *New England Journal of Medicine* did not lead, as hoped, to widespread acceptance and use of tPA or even, in some quarters, to acknowledgment that it worked. This was not because the effect of the drug was minimal or ambiguous—quite the contrary. But critics emerged among stroke doctors, neurologists, and emergency physicians. Although stroke was a devastating and frequently lethal disease, critics sniped about possible harm and questioned the extent of benefit, even though the NINDS treatment effect was substantially greater than what can be demonstrated for most medicines. The NINDS investigators would be perplexed, angered, and disappointed.

"In cancer," said Pat Lyden, "if a group of young researchers had found a treatment that reduced the disability burden by 50% as we did, they would be carried into meetings in sedan chairs."

Instead of acceptance there followed rancorous disputes in neurology, then refusal and denial among emergency physicians. Ignorance would be sown in the field of health care generally and would persist among the wider public. The conflict lasted years, and in some quarters it has not ended yet. In an ideal world, tPA could be used annually in the United States alone to treat some 400,000 patients—roughly half of stroke victims. Even one-third that number—a realistic goal—would make a huge difference in terms of adult disability.

To understand why so few know about tPA even today, and why so many doctors do not learn how or when to use it, the NINDS study itself is the place to start. Its leaders and investigators—many of whom have gone on to become well-known academic physicians—defend and laud its accomplishments while acknowledging the controversies. No question but it stands as a watershed.

At the same time, in attempting to make the study definitive, it is fair to say that its leaders overshot the mark. Twenty-two months after patient recruitment began, in early 1993, hoping for a "consistent and persuasive" result—which, in fact, they already possessed—the study's administrative leaders decided to continue and expand it rather than to conclude it and publish the results. As a consequence, they sat on strongly positive data for more than 2 years, and in the end this stratagem did not yield the response they hoped for, much less the appreciation for persistence and thoroughness that in so many respects they all deserved. True, hindsight is perfect. But in extending the study and chopping it in two, they may have unwittingly contributed to the chilly reception accorded tPA for stroke after FDA approval finally came in June 1996. How this happened is a cautionary tale that speaks to the wisdom of procedural transparency in science, no matter the best of intentions.

In 1978, when Michael Walker was hired to head the stroke division at NINDS, he found exactly one clinical trial under way. True, as a branch of the National Institutes of Health (NIH), NINDS was heavily invested in basic research. Clinically, there was emphasis on prevention; but as to treatment, the prevailing sentiment among senior neurologists was simple: there was nothing much to be done. Walker, who had run brain tumor trials at the National Cancer Institute, did not share this pervasive attitude of defeatism. A neurosurgeon by training, he was inclined to fix things. An experienced administrator, visiting the various outside institutions funded by NINDS, Walker was dismayed: "None of the basic research had a translational aspect into what is good in the clinic."

To counter the inertia of pessimism, Walker set in motion a new research methodology, which he called the Task Order Master Agreement. The aim was to promote preliminary studies for stroke treatments. Any that hinted at success, he hoped, would provoke in turn the larger phase III trials that the FDA relies upon as proving (or not) the worth of candidate drugs. Walker imported the Task Order concept from his work in cancer research: NINDS would accredit institutions able and willing to conduct clinical trials and contract with researchers to carry them out. At the same time NINDS would serve as a conduit by which pharmaceutical firms could supply drugs for research and, in return, at no further cost, harvest reliable data.

Walker laid it down from the beginning that although drug company scientists were welcome to contribute insight, their marketing people were not. Further, study data would be published, favorable or not. After several firms took up the offer, one early result was the NIH Stroke Scale. The most recent of several instruments to assess severity, this 42-point scale continues to be widely used to evaluate patients—in 3 to 5 minutes—for tPA.

To develop and manage trials, Walker hired John Marler. A tall, lanky Colorado-born physician fresh from a neurology residency at the Mayo Clinic, his background included community organizing. A graduate of West Virginia University Medical School, he had worked for the Volunteers in Service to America (VISTA)—the domestic equivalent of the Peace Corps—making his decision to work for the government a logical career move.

Marler came to NINDS already interested in clot-busting agents. He was not alone. As he familiarized himself with current research, he could see a number of people had arrived at the same conclusion independently. Despite the failed trials with streptokinase in the 1960s, the new agents—most notably tPA—held promise. In 1980 the NIH had circulated a consensus statement that absolutely contraindicated thrombolytic therapy for stroke. That view, just 4 years later, might well be in need of revision.

Zivin met John Marler in 1985, shortly before his paper appeared in *Science* and soon after he started reviewing grant proposals at the NIH. Katherine Woodbury Harris, a grants-review scientist at NINDS who knew of Marler's interest in thrombolysis for stroke, suggested they talk. They lunched together, discussed prospects for clinical trials with tPA, and remained afterward in frequent contact. Marler would use the rabbit stroke model to advance a basis for human studies, and he promoted funding for Zivin's ongoing research.

What crystallized for Marler as he worked his way through the literature was the factor that turned out to be of utmost significance: time-to-treatment. He came across, in particular, a recent paper from Harvard's neurosurgery laboratory that suggested, on evidence from experiments with monkeys, that 3 hours of an occluded cerebral vessel might be the upper limit for avoiding permanent brain damage. Zivin, who learned of this work from a collaborator, Umberto DeGirolami of the Harvard group, would eventually re-analyze the data to statistically extract from those experiments the strong relationship between duration of ischemia and magnitude of infarct. In individual cases, predicting partial or complete recovery based on time was not possible; strokes were too variable. But one could reliably determine that in people most strokes were complete—maximum damage inflicted—within 6 hours. For purposes of clinical trials, the ideal time-to-treatment would be about 100 minutes. Shorter timeframes would mean dispensing the drug to some patients who would spontaneously recover in any event, while longer times would make them less likely to benefit.

The real-world ramification, Marler reasoned, was to incorporate time as a factor in clinical trials in a disciplined way. For the use of thrombolysis in heart attack, cardiologists were also developing an appreciation of what became known as "door-to-needle time." With stroke the danger of disability made urgency even greater. Patients in the older, failed research with streptokinase had been treated many hours and even days after first signs and symptoms. That would have to change in future trials.

So in 1985, when Marler first began to envision clinical studies of tPA, he built into the protocol (the rules for conducting trials) strict adherence to a short time window. From his own experience working and hanging around emergency rooms as a VISTA volunteer, and again at the Mayo Clinic, he had seen first-hand how physicians simply tended to let a stroke run its course. The ischemic stroke patient, helpless and unhelped in the emergency suite, "needed a friend," as he put it. For the incipient NINDS-supported studies, time was to become brain. He decided upon treatment as imperative within 1 hour—lengthened for practical reasons to 90 minutes.

"You can't imagine how crazy the idea of treating stroke within 60 minutes of the onset of symptoms was considered by most neurologists," recalls Marler. "It was considered foolhardy and foolish and impossible." Indeed, when neurologist Tom Brott and two colleagues learned that NINDS was about to let contracts for pilot studies with tPA, they were astounded by the proposed time-frame: 90 minutes sounded totally unreasonable. Meeting with Walker and Marler, Brott remembers: "We thought we would be able to convince them to treat patients within 4 hours, which we thought was something we could do." But no such luck: "They would not have anything to do with that. They were insistent that patients be treated within 90 minutes."

Brott, then assistant professor of neurology at the University of Cincinnati, nevertheless accepted the proposed contract, as did colleagues David Levy from Cornell University and E. Clarke Haley at the University of Virginia.

Also doubtful, albeit sympathetic, to the short time-to-treatment was Elliott Grossbard of Genentech. Marler had asked the company to supply tPA for trials. After writing a letter and hearing nothing, he turned to Burroughs Wellcome, the British firm that was testing its own version of the drug; he was in talks with them when Grossbard showed up at his office, unannounced.

Genentech had decided to provide the drug, after all. Among company executives, concern about stroke apparently abated. Zivin, although he had no interaction with Grossbard, had become an adviser to Genentech scientists after publication of the *Science* paper, and his work may have helped shift the weight of opinion (see Chapter 5). He knew he had convinced at least Bill Bennett, one of the company's chief scientists, who led the tPA research team, that the drug was likely to be safe and effective for stroke just as for heart attack. But concern remained, not unreasonably at the time, that tPA could provoke hemorrhage as an adverse effect.

"The reason we're giving it to you is we don't think you'll be able to do it as fast as you say," Marler recalls Grossbard telling him, adding, "I want you to know that this is the most potent drug that anyone has ever used.... I want you to be very careful."

Although the concept of the randomized controlled trial (RCT) may be traced back about a thousand years, only in the past half-century has it become the solid and reliable standard for evaluating new therapies. Its importance is due to the "chemotherapeutic revolution" that began in the 1950s, when ever-more-powerful drugs demanded regulatory attention. Anchored in statistical analysis, such well-designed trials are often long and always expensive, but they usually yield trustworthy results. Able to address a wide range of serious and complex disorders, RCTs in the United States aim both to demonstrate that a drug works and to satisfy the FDA that it is safe to manufacture, market, and prescribe. The relatively large "phase III" studies are generally preceded by "phase I" and "phase II" studies that seek to discover an appropriate safe dose for the drug that is at least potentially therapeutic, and a satisfactory way to administer it.

So for tPA for stroke, the early pilot studies tried to find the proper dose and also aimed to demonstrate that time-to-treatment within 90 minutes was feasible. Tom Brott, especially, took the challenge to treat fast as an opportunity to innovate; he is credited with creating a model that became widely emulated during the NINDS study. Cell phones were not in wide use in 1986, but they existed: big clunky appliances mostly used in cars and trucks. They were becoming more common now that the Federal Communications Commission had allocated special mobile frequencies. Brott recognized that in terms of response time, this technology could improve on the paging system then in use, by which a doctor equipped with a "beeper" would go to a regular phone after receiving a signal and a number to call.

"We would get a page from an emergency department and not answer it but get into our car," recalls Brott. Driving to the hospital, the doctor would call the pharmacy, emergency room, and CT scanner. "We were able to treat patients within 90 minutes primarily by using cellular phone technology and a multi-hospital network." It was "parallel processing, where you're doing everything at once."

In addition, the way Brott and his colleagues worked made them welcome in all the Cincinnati area hospitals. They attended to every emergency stroke whether tPA could be used or not. At the time the FDA had just approved the drug for heart attack, so its profile was strongly positive. Emergency room doctors and nurses were familiar with it and could readily learn how to admit stroke patients, enroll them, and "push" the drug—by intravenous injection followed by a slow drip. Moreover, these early phase I studies were "open label."

That meant all personnel involved knew they were giving tPA; there was no mystery, as there would be with a placebo-controlled trial. "So you'd go to the emergency room, meet with a very friendly reception," recalls Brott, "almost without exception."

The first of two pilot studies eventually recruited 73 patients for treatment in under 90 minutes, but some 732 patients had to be evaluated to reach that number. A second, smaller study included a second "arm" in which some patients were treated inside 3 hours. From these trials emerged a plausible dosage—considerably lower than that used with heart attack—and clear validation for the idea that tPA could be administered within such a short timeframe. How well or badly it worked with ischemic stroke remained to be quantified, however. The results offered clear hints of success but nothing definitive. Finally, a third small study was not open label but randomized, controlled, and blinded. All three together delivered a single message: "Clearly, additional larger, placebo-controlled trials of rt-PA therapy in early acute stroke are needed."

Now from Mike Walker came a critical decision—to have NINDS run the next step, the larger randomized study. Originally he had envisaged the government organization as running only preliminary clinical studies. The longer and more difficult trials that enrolled many more patients, he expected, would be conducted under other auspices—most often by a team at one or more medical centers. But tPA, with its special potential, in his view warranted exceptional attention. It "looked interesting and promising enough, and complex enough, I felt that the institute should fund [the trial] independently, and we should run it." As head of the stroke division, he approached NINDS executives and requested funds for just such a purpose. "I thought this was the way I could push the field of stroke and cerebrovascular disease further ahead, if we could just learn something about how you treat these people."

Thus was conceived the NINDS Stroke Study. Technically, it would be a large phase IIB trial with multiple medical centers participating, with a phase III trial to follow if warranted.*

As project director and team leader, John Marler would attend to the trial on a day-to-day basis. He saw to setting up the various committees: executive, steering, drug distribution. A Coordinating Center located at Henry Ford

---

*The "phases" in FDA terminology are terms of art, not strictly defined. Generally speaking phase II trials, larger than phase I trials, provide the opportunity to eliminate unpromising candidates and gauge prospects for promising drugs by making it possible to develop definitive protocols in preparation for phase III studies. While phase IIA trials are usually concerned with issues of dosage, phase IIB trials are concerned with showing both efficacy and safety and so resemble phase III trials.

Hospital in Detroit would collect the data and report to the FDA on any dangerous side effects. There was—as in most large studies—a Data and Safety Monitoring Committee (DSMC), a five-person panel to provide a further level of protection for patients and to avoid investigator bias. In an unusual and questionable move, Mike Walker himself initially chaired the DSMC. (A rule of trial design is that members of the DSMC should all be independent of the administrators and participants that run the clinical trial.)

To decide on participating institutions, Marler chose from among some 70-odd applicants. After a review panel scored them, contracts were let finally to nine—later eight—most of them large urban medical centers affiliated with other metropolitan hospitals and universities. In part because African-Americans are at higher risk for stroke, Marler made an effort to include hospitals where minorities would and could be recruited.

Marler worked out the basic protocol for the study in conjunction with the investigators. Time-to-treatment would be 90 minutes for half the patients and 3 hours for the other half. Treating strokes fast could represent a new paradigm for future studies, and Marler himself actually would have preferred the 90-minute window for all, but Mike Walker insisted he add a 3-hour arm.

Viewed in retrospect, the rapid treatment concept positively shaped not just drug delivery but the makeup and character of the entire study. The local principal investigators were, by and large, younger neurologists. Attracted to this new emergency model, unlike many senior colleagues they were willing to put up with years of inconvenience and disruption in their professional and personal lives. Older doctors, often accustomed to writing their own rules and submitting grant applications, seem to have shied away from the study, with its unprecedented demands on their time. However, granting the temerity of youth, had experienced physicians worked outside NINDS to organize their own trial and followed the usual vetting process, later problematic decisions might have been minimized or avoided. Indeed from the standpoint of scientific methodology and clinical trials design, there were issues of decision-making, authority, and transparency to the NINDS study that are disconcerting.

Rapid response also demanded local solutions. The system Tom Brott had invented in Cincinnati was adaptable, but with some 40 hospitals and medical centers, situations varied. Barbara Tilley, after she was selected as principal investigator and chief statistician of the Coordinating Center, traveled to every facility and walked through the reception of acute stroke patients. At one medical center in New York, the tPA stretcher for speeding patients to the CT scanning suite was chained to the wall so as to always have it ready. At another hospital, to avoid a slow-running elevator nurses would cover the patient with a blanket for transport across a parking lot to a newer building.

"Every emergency department," said Tilley, "was like getting to know a person. What their idiosyncracies were and what you had to do."

Tilley and Welch did not just observe; they helped hospitals make stroke care fast and efficient. Welch relied on quality improvement measures associated with W. Edwards Deming, who had first brought statistical control methods in manufacturing to Japan and, by the 1980s, to the United States—all undergirded by a philosophy of efficiency and quality. "We drew up Deming charts and had improvement committees," said Welch. The concept of Total Quality Improvement was enjoying a vogue in health care. "There are pros and cons to that system, but it certainly worked in getting recruitment in."

The first patients in the NINDS Stroke Study were enrolled and treated in January 1991.

Among themselves the local principal investigators began calling tPA "Brain-O" after the product for clearing clogged pipes. Whether it worked for stroke they did not yet know, but over the next 4 years they developed *esprit du corps* and a durable camaraderie. Sometimes self-described as "young Turks," they met fairly frequently. "There was a real bonding among the investigators who worked on the trial," said Steve Horowitz, who was not a stroke specialist but a general neurologist and had completed fellowship training in neuromuscular disorders. Older than most, he worked at Long Island Jewish Medical Center, a New York metropolitan institution that straddles the Borough of Queens at the Nassau county line, crisscrossed by busy highways. He felt himself a bit of an outsider at first, but the stroke doctors "could not have been more welcoming and respectful."

For some, the emergency aspect and demanding protocol must have resonated with the chronic stresses of residency and internship. But what really attracted them and cemented them as a group was the prospect of proving a powerful drug for an untreatable disease. Steve Levine, who went on to become a professor of neurology, first at Mount Sinai School of Medicine and more recently at SUNY Downstate Medical Center, joked that if it weren't for the NINDS study, "I'd probably be playing chess in Central Park."

Pat Lyden, at the University of California San Diego (UCSD), was still a resident when Zivin had arrived in 1985. UCSD had not been his first choice, but his girlfriend insisted—then promptly ended their relationship. But Lyden came to like the school and exchanged his plans to become a neurosurgeon in favor of clinical neurology and research. Lyden became Zivin's first fellow at UCSD. When contracts were being let for the NINDS trials, they applied: "Whether because of Zivin's reputation or because of the fact that I was known as a wild-haired crazy guy, for whatever reason, we got the contract."

But among San Diego doctors, Zivin and Lyden did not enjoy the welcoming spirit Tom Brott had nurtured in Cincinnati. When they asked local physicians for help in facilitating and publicizing emergency treatment for stroke, recalled Lyden, "They literally laughed at us." During a classic evening at the medical society, "They said, 'This is insane. You guys need to do your research on prisoners.'"

Nevertheless, Lyden became one of the most active and aggressive stroke doctors in the study. He felt himself in competition with Tom Brott in Cincinnati and Jim Grotta at the University of Texas in Houston, and made it his goal that UCSD enroll the most patients. When John Rothrock, the other leading clinical stroke neurologist at UCSD, decided to see only patients who made their way to the university emergency rooms, Lyden secured staff privileges at five other area hospitals. He gained the cooperation of ER personnel and put himself on call 24 hours a day, 7 days a week.

"I had my car equipped with an illegal siren and illegal high beams and I had a light on top of the car." For 4 years he would run red lights and drive on the shoulder of the freeway: "Whatever I had to do to get to these hospitals." Traffic patterns in sprawling San Diego were not amenable to Deming's Total Quality Improvement, and reaching the metropolitan hospitals via streets and highways that cut through hill and dale around the coastal city proved a challenge. The team at the University of Cincinnati eventually added 150 cases to the NINDS study; at UCSD, 146. Each evaluated five times as many patients.

The study's objective: Did tPA for stroke work? Was it safe and effective? Nothing better showed the value of an RCT than the issues surrounding sudden improvement and cerebral hemorrhage—the former highly desirable, the latter a potential disaster.

Typically tPA worked fast. But in most cases, hours if not days and weeks would pass before patients were fully normal or had maximally recovered from deficits. Occasionally a patient would improve dramatically and suddenly. In the NINDS study, recalls Lyden, "We were seeing these on-the-table responses—these 'oh, wow!' responses—and [some of us] thought we were seeing a great drug." The Lazarus phenomenon, it was sometimes called, after the biblical beggar raised from the dead.

Both Zivin and Lyden had encountered this kind of response to tPA outside the NINDS study, and it could be gratifying but unnerving. Zivin had participated in a dose-finding trial that used a competing form of tPA, tested briefly by Burroughs Wellcome. One day a 70-year-old man was helicoptered to UCSD with a severe stroke. Awakening from a brief nap, he had been unable to move one side of his body and was completely aphasic—unable to talk. Consent obtained, he was injected with tPA. An angiogram performed before and after the drug was given revealed that the clot had indeed dissolved. When Zivin entered the radiology suite, the patient lay draped and inert on the examination table. Zivin said to the nurses, "Thank you." From the patient, invisible beneath the sheet and mass of towels, came a hair-raising echo: *"Thank you."*

Lyden's potentially career-wrecking story happened just before the NINDS trial started. A young woman, just 34 years old and shortly to be married, endured a week of migraine headaches before feeling well enough to go shopping with her mother for bridesmaids' gowns. But at the department store she went into the bathroom and did not come out. Moments later her mother found her there, lying on the floor. She was completely paralyzed on the left side, blind, numb, and generally unresponsive. Her doctor, a colleague of Lyden's in private practice, phoned him.

Should she receive tPA?

Lyden told the doctor to go ahead, to use the proper dose; he would meet them at the hospital. But on arriving he discovered that his physician friend seemed stalled, apparently too fearful to start the treatment. Lyden himself took charge and a nurse, Traci Babcock, administered the tPA.

"I had never done this on a human before," recalled Lyden. "I had treated plenty of rabbits."

No sooner was the tPA injected than it occurred to him that he was in a hospital where he had no privileges and consequently was not covered for malpractice. The woman's fiancé had introduced himself: he was a lawyer. About 30 minutes later the patient said loudly: "Oh, my God—my head!" Headache in a stroke victim is a frequent sign of hemorrhage.

Lyden rushed the patient for a CT scan, fully expecting to find a big bleed, but the picture came back normal. Then he noticed the patient was holding her head with her *left* hand, which had been paralyzed moments before.

"The next day she was moving everything normally. Her sensory deficit was almost completely resolved and her vision was normal."

Despite such experiences, there was no telling. Intuition sometimes proved misleading. In San Diego at least, after results were revealed, patients were informed as to whether they had received tPA or a placebo. Doctors were often enough surprised.

Similarly, the issue of bleeding strokes preoccupied the NINDS researchers from beginning to end. Ischemic strokes turning into hemorrhagic strokes had been the downfall of streptokinase. In general, many strokes—an estimated one in five—start as ischemic events but subsequently undergo what is known as hemorrhagic conversion or transformation. For the study, the question was whether tPA added to the risk of symptomatic hemorrhage and could therefore foment more harm than good.

Here fears and impressions also proved no guide. Mike Welch, responsible for the overall conduct of the trial, investigated every hemorrhage. As it happened, the very first case recruited for the trial turned into a bleeding stroke. "It was with a sinking feeling," recalled Welch, "that we reviewed that case. Because we thought if every one was going to be like this, we're in real trouble." But nothing like that happened. He was blinded to the treatment—whether the patient had been treated with drug or placebo. But the DSMC was not, and every three hemorrhages brought about a long look at the clinical situation in each case and scrutiny of the study as a whole. In the end, there was a 6% increase in symptomatic hemorrhage in patients who received tPA but no net increase in mortality. The issue of hemorrhage is discussed more fully in Chapter 6, but to anticipate: The incidence of severe toxicity actually due to tPA, recalculated from the original NINDS data, is today put at about 1–3%, an altogether acceptable risk in a therapy for a frequently fatal and potentially devastating disease.

After 18 months of adequately paced recruitment, by the fall of 1992 the NINDS Stroke Study was nearing its original goal of 280 randomized patients. Then, for reasons that remain to this day clouded by shifting intentions, vagaries of drug regulation, half-perceived danger of harm, and perhaps even the persistent and insidious impact of therapeutic nihilism—for some combination of reasons such as these, the NINDS administrators moved the goal posts. The study did not end; the data were not analyzed or published in good order.

In retrospect, the weighty decision to continue and extend the NINDS study would not help tPA win easy acceptance once approved to treat acute stroke; if anything, it made it more difficult. Had the original Phase IIB Study concluded in a timely way, been analyzed and published, the result might have been more rapid FDA endorsement and gradual but non-controversial acceptance by the various stakeholders—neurologists, emergency physicians, and hospitals. Subsequent accounts by the NINDS study administrators and investigators do not examine the advantages to this more normative route. Why did it happen the way it did? Misperceptions around the FDA approval process, practical considerations about complex trials, and paradoxical concerns over potential ethical issues—each of these played a role.

Front and center in this story is the wisdom and basis for conducting a second trial before exposing the results of the first. As Mike Walker explains it, the FDA required for drug approval two large separate trials that each demonstrated efficacy. "They at the time had the concept that they wanted two completely independent controlled, prospective, randomized trials demonstrating efficacy, and one was not sufficient." This view was by no means Walker's alone. It was shared by John Marler, members of the DSMC and, probably in consequence, many of the investigators associated with the study. But it was based on long-standing practice rather than any formal rule—and it was wrong.

The requirement for a second trial, in fact, would partly owe to how convincing were the results of the first trial. The *P*-value, which represents the probability that the difference between treatment and placebo is due to chance, is a quantitative measure of success. By convention, a P-value of .05 or under—less is better—indicates a positive outcome, with about 5/100ths or a 1-in-20 possibility that success is a result of chance. A second trial would likely be called for. But with a much more powerful *P*-value, such as tPA achieved (.001 for the global outcome in the NINDS trial), another trial was arguably neither logical nor required. The odds were not more than 1 in 1000 that the results were due to chance.[†]

In addition, there was precedence. By 1991 several powerful drugs—notably to treat kidney failure and neutropenia (low white blood cell count)—had been approved on the basis of a single Phase III study. Devices were typically approved on the basis of one trial. And the FDA, at the instigation of the George H. W. Bush administration, had also announced in 1991 that it would use flexibility "whenever possible to measure the efficacy of drugs used to treat life-threatening diseases."

The move toward a plan to bypass the normal route, which would have been to simply analyze and publish the results of the trial, began to unfold in late 1992. Walker and other members of the DSMC examined the results, first for the primary endpoint, and they seem to have been at once dismayed and encouraged. In any event, they called a meeting.

"We had a situation," recounts Pat Lyden, "after 300 patients when the DSMC said, you have to stop. We have a problem, something we got to talk about. But they wouldn't tell us what it was. And they said there was a data issue."

Lyden recalls being perplexed. He was summoned to testify. He and E. Clarke Haley were to represent the investigators.

"Did that mean we had a harm issue? Or did it mean we had succeeded? Or did it mean something else? We didn't know what it meant."

Lyden's questions were to the point. In any trial the DSMC has two oversight functions: to stop a trial if the drug being tested is causing harm, or to end a trial if it is a clear success. In both cases the aim is to protect patients. With the NINDS study, the DSMC was about to overstep these customary boundaries.

The December 1992 meeting in Bethesda, Maryland, took place, as Lyden remembers it, in "this dive, almost a Motel 6." Although its minutes do not

---

[†]In clinical trials the *P* value represents the probability that a result indicating a difference between the treatment and placebo is due to chance.

allude to grim surroundings, they do convey a sense of grave concern. In executive session, Mike Walker began by noting the "extraordinary complexity and sensitivity of the issues to be discussed." It was becoming ever more difficult to justify further double-blind randomized trials with tPA, he said, which was already approved for heart attack and, from the way the data was shaping up, looking favorable for stroke.

So rather than consider how the data from the study would be cleaned up and analyzed—as would happen under ordinary circumstances—the DSMC discussed continuing and expanding the study. The "data issue" turned out to be the study's "primary endpoint," which for success had been set as a 4-point improvement on the NIH Stroke Scale in tPA-treated patients at 24 hours. This endpoint was actually not designed to test efficacy but only to show whether the drug was having a positive short-term impact. Of course, there was no choosing after the fact. "You had to pick a single outcome," Walker emphasized years later, "and you had to power and sample size your trial in order to achieve that outcome, and you lived or died by that single outcome." Ambiguous numbers around the 24-hour endpoint would later turn out to be a trivial, but it gave the trial a technically negative outcome.

What was to be done? Echoing Walker, as the project officer running the trial on a daily basis, John Marler suggested that recent publications "were making it progressively more difficult to continue a double-blind placebo controlled study." As a result, "protocol modification," he said, was already under discussion with representatives at the FDA. One suggestion—no one seems to know where it came from—was that the trial could continue to recruit more patients and simply increase its sample size while changing the problematic primary endpoint. But this was an unlikely solution just because, as Marler later noted, it would be "kind of against all the rules of clinical trials."

Not surprisingly, a project officer at the FDA, Rebecca Dachman, "came to us with a flat no" to that idea.

But Marler presented either Dachman's own suggestion or the one that she had adopted after talks with him and others: she "told us to just divide the trial in two." Dachman suggested "that we just keep the same protocol with a change in the endpoints, sample size, and patient treatment."

With this proposed change on the table, Pat Lyden and E. Clarke Haley testified on behalf of the local principal investigators.

Lyden told the DSMC: "We're all committed to this, we're putting our heart and soul into it. But if we're hurting people you need to tell us."

Being constantly oncall, treating patients with tPA or placebo or not at all, and constant concern about hemorrhage carried personal and professional costs. As Lyden later noted, he was now divorced and other marriages were not prospering, either. Stress, not just on the academic doctors but on the nurses and other personnel, ought not to go ignored. But Lyden also said, "If we're close, don't stop us. We want to see this thing through." In turn, Haley presented the DSMC with a written statement of the investigators' "interests, concerns, worries, and needs."

After hearing this testimony and taking a report from Barbara Tilley and Mike Welch of the Coordinating Center, the DSMC retired into closed session. Members seem to have entertained the possibility that "the investigators could stop their original study, complete follow-up of all patients, and analyze and publish the results of their activity study as designed." But they rejected this in favor of the FDA-endorsed suggestion to continue the study, enlarge it, and recruit patients for a second trial. They subsequently presented "comments and recommendations" that would be better characterized as a set of top-down directives. At the end of the meeting, the DSMC delivered a message that, at the time, Lyden remembered, seemed "quite mysterious."

The investigators were instructed to enroll 300 more patients—an order that would take a couple of more years to fulfill. The aim, as they were told, was to discover whether tPA for acute stroke could provide a "clear and persuasive" benefit.

"And we had no idea what that meant," recalls Lyden.

The panel told them not to question its decision among themselves or to talk with anyone else about it. The panel reassured them "that their concerns about safety, the protection of patients, and the practicality of continued investigation have been fully taken into account." They were thanked for their hard work and dedication.

The NINDS study now restarted to proceed essentially as before. The only change was the primary endpoint, which for the second trial was designated as post-stroke evaluation at 90 days. The same centers, the same personnel, the same protocols. Only the primary endpoint would change. This second trial would be a twin of the first in every respect except name: it would be called a "pivotal" Phase III study.‡ Several months later, NINDS brought investigators and statisticians together in a workshop that aimed to design a convincing measure of the study's success. Their solution was a "global test" that would combine the various measures used to assess stroke patients—the Barthel Index, Modified Rankin Scale, Glasgow Outcome Scale, and National Institutes

---

‡Sponsors and the FDA frequently categorize certain trials as "pivotal." These are trials meant to conclusively demonstrate the efficacy and safety of a drug for its proposed indication and provide the best information for clinical decision-making. Pivotal trials are typically Phase III trials, but again there is no formal definition.

of Health Stroke Scale. In the event, their sophisticated and well-meaning effort was not really necessary because in the final analysis all four measures would turn out to be highly positive.

"We ran what were essentially two sequential trials," explained Mike Walker, "ran one after the other, split seamlessly in the middle." He would claim a substantial advantage because the group of investigators already in place could "move the trial right along."

In fact, although the NINDS stroke trials would prove a rare success, the road to completion now became unduly long. The last patient was not randomized until October 1994, and results of the first trial would only be revealed a year after that, when the celebrated NINDS study was published in *The New England Journal of Medicine*.

Study leaders, that is to say, sat on strongly positive data for 2 years and more—despite the fact that tPA was available in every emergency room in the country. In the mid-1990s, tPA for heart attack, approved in 1987, was hitting its stride nationwide—a situation that would eventually change with the growing popularity of new device-based procedures, notably angioplasty and stents. The delay of many months in reporting the results of the NINDS trials, whether or not it substantially impeded the reception of tPA for stroke, certainly did not help. In terms of normal science, the breach with customary research procedures was difficult to justify. The best that can be said is that clinical trials are human endeavors and no randomized controlled trial is perfect.

Not surprisingly, the local principal investigators supported the call to extend the trial. They had bonded as a group, worked under the authority of the NINDS administrators, and were doctors who would not abandon their peers. They were not expert in the operations and procedures of the FDA, and their perspective on the NINDS study remained in place even 15 years later. The various rationales for dividing the study into two trials became part of its standard lore. Said Lyden: "The [DSMC] did an incredibly courageous thing, which was to make us keep going. Because in the end we ended up with two 300-patient studies, both of which showed benefit. And the FDA took those two studies and approved the drug."

Zivin disagreed with this assessment. On an organizational basis, he faulted the DSMC for arrogating authority to itself and the investigators for allowing it to happen. Given the importance of the study, it was as if the umpires of the World Series suddenly started to manage the players. Most of all, he viewed the continuation of the NINDS study and the long delay in announcing and publishing the results as unacceptable. Earlier approval might have meant less controversy, more ready and growing acceptance and, over the ensuing years, treatment for potentially hundreds of thousands of stroke victims.

But no sooner had he voiced his objections to Mike Walker, as the initial trial came to end, than he was asked to leave the study, ostensibly for a conflict of interest. (Zivin provides a first-person account in a separate statement at the end of this book). Not involved in the day-to-day recruitment of patients, he had left the clinical territory to Pat Lyden and John Rothrock while he tended to the more basic research for which he was funded. The arrangement, to which he agreed but did not like much himself, may have lent distance and perspective to his viewpoint. In his view, the fact that the "primary endpoint" of improvement at 24 hours failed to reach statistical significance was in itself of no importance; it was an artifact of study design unconnected to the substance of the results, and the FDA, he contended, would have recognized as much. With the drug already approved for heart attack, FDA administrators could have called on a panel of experts—as they did often enough when warranted—to independently review the data and to make recommendations and then act accordingly. In this way, tPA for stroke could have been approved more than 2 years earlier than it was.

Finally, what about the FDA? In general, clinical trials administrators consult with the organization and may request advice as to trial design. To this end Mike Walker and John Marler were assigned Rebecca Dachman, who worked in the Clinical Trials Branch. She was a physician who worked at the FDA's Center for Biologics Evaluation and Research (CBER), a division created in 1988 from the old public health service that for decades had regulated vaccines and blood banks. Its mission was to evaluate the new products emerging from advanced biotech such as recombinant drugs like tPA.

How Dachman came to her recommendations for the NINDS study remains unclear. One should add, of course, that Dachman's advisory role was only that. If Marler and Walker had disagreed with her conclusions and recommendations, there were several levels of appeal and, if a supervisory assessment failed, recourse to a review panel of experts would be another option.

But in the event, not until that morning at Airlie in August 1995, when Barbara Tilley sent up the results on overhead projectors to reveal the numbers to the investigators, did the three dozen researchers erupt in cheers. Long ago in America it was common to drink spirits before lunch, and on that day in August, ante-meridian Champagne flowed once more.

Mike Welch recalled his feeling of "absolute complete joy" in recognizing "that this was a major moment, the first time ever that anything had proved to be effective in acute stroke."

After some revelry and a review of the data, the group divided into committees that worked all weekend on a paper to explain and analyze the study.

Barbara Tilley provided each of the participants with a booklet that detailed the results, with extensive cross-tabulation of statistics. Collectively they drafted the article that John Marler would refine over the next several months.

Not until publication of "Tissue Plasminogen Activator for Acute Ischemic Stroke" in the *New England Journal of Medicine* in December 1995 would the public learn of the study's success. NINDS called a major press conference that brought study administrators and local principal investigators before the major news organizations. Pat Lyden felt like a Mercury astronaut, and the whole affair was straight out of *The Right Stuff*: "And you just know you're in a moment that's a paradigm change."

That sensation of participating in something historic was widespread and even extended to the big bottle of Mad Dog wine that nobody drank that day at Airlie. Barbara Tilley took it home unopened and for years afterward kept it on a shelf in her office. But eventually someone wondered aloud if she were an alcoholic, so she took it down.

Tilley also noted, reflecting on it years later, that tPA represented a new paradigm. As a convenient way to describe a thoroughgoing shift in treatment strategy, so it did. And like many new paradigms—in medicine, especially any brand of new that imposes upon habit and practice and traditional comportment—it provoked both favorable reception but also dismay and resistance. Here was tPA at last, the first effective treatment ever for acute stroke. And its troubles had just begun.

Part | 2

Change, Resistance, and Transformation

The Brain Doctors Cometh—Slowly | 5

"If I'm driving through your town in the next few years, and I'm brought into your emergency room with a stroke," said Don Easton, rising to speak at a meeting soon after the NINDS results were presented, "Would you please remember: 72 milligrams?" He was referring to the dose of tPA, prepared for individuals based on body weight. Easton, at 175 pounds or 80 kilos, added: "And give it as fast as you can."

Easton, who had chaired the Data Safety and Monitoring Committee for the second half of the NINDS study, was surprised by the cold reception for tPA. In spite of any negatives that detractors wanted to put up, the results were clear as a bell and, as he said, "So let's get on with treatment." Most if not all of the NINDS study researchers were equally taken aback.

"We thought this would be welcome, open arms welcome," recalled Steve Levine. "It was just 180 degrees opposite. It was like, 'This is too dangerous, and we don't believe it.'"

At first, to be sure, there was a spark of bright promise. Soon after the results appeared in the *New England Journal of Medicine* in late 1995, Genentech made its case for FDA approval. The drug sailed through that often drawn-out process inside 6 months. Although Genentech was to barely advertise the drug for stroke, tPA was already widely available in hospital pharmacies and would henceforth carry a new label with the new indication in addition to heart disease and pulmonary embolism. In addition, two big organizations, the American Academy of Neurology and the American Heart Association, both moved quickly to endorse it. At NINDS, Mike Walker and John Marler planned a public information program.

Inasmuch as there had never been a treatment for stroke, one would have to wonder, in view of the 11% to 13% *absolute* benefit, why a doctor would not wish to use it. True, with any drug some physicians will be early adopters and others, with concern for unforeseen adverse effects, are more cautious. Nevertheless, as a one-time intervention for a serious and common disease, tPA more resembled a surgical procedure with excellent results and only a slight but acceptable risk of harm. The NINDS study had also shown tPA did not increase either mortality or the number of patients with grave physical and mental deficits; it did not save people from death only to leave them hopelessly disabled.

But then came the cold water: doubt, disbelief, skepticism. Resistance was greatly complicated by exaggerated concern over cerebral hemorrhage. Now began the most contentious debate over a drug ever seen in neurology.

In retrospect, it should not have been quite so surprising, for tPA was a demanding drug, just as stroke was a hyper-acute condition. Its emergency protocol, CT scan, and individualized dosing could make it laborious. If neurologists accepted the NINDS results, they would be in effect required to change both the way they perceived stroke and how they treated it. Fine to call it a revolutionary pharmaceutical—but revolutions are not always or even usually popular, at least at first. Although some leading specialists had been saying for about 10 years that stroke should be treated in its acute phase, what was the urgency when nothing could be done besides make a diagnosis? Now tPA threatened to change all that. Neurologists were accustomed to an office practice. They were not anxious to be torn away from their desks or roused to the hospital in the middle of the night. They should now become emergency responders? They did not like it.

At first not even stroke specialists could agree. In mid-1996, a few months after the *New England Journal of Medicine* article was published, a thrombolysis meeting took place in Copenhagen. Everybody showed up. Gregory del Zoppo helped organize it. Désiré Collen, whose work had pioneered the whole field, was there; also NINDS study researchers John Marler, Tom Brott, Jim Grotta, and Pat Lyden, among others. Importantly, tPA skeptics attended, including Louis R. Caplan and Anthony Furlan. During presentations and in the corridors during the meeting, tPA was frequently discussed with respect to the upcoming FDA meeting that would rule on the drug.

Ethics entered the picture: that was the intriguing thing. Furlan, for one, questioned whether the NINDS trial really provided enough information.

He wanted to know, as he wrote in a paper that appeared in 1997, "under what current circumstances we can justify exposing ischemic stroke patients to an increased acute risk of hemorrhage and death from thrombolysis." (The NINDS trial did not report an increased risk of death, in fact; this was an inference on Furlan's part.) And was the "consistent" benefit reported for tPA with all types of stroke "precise enough to justify individual patient treatment decisions?" Dealing with patients of all ages and severity of stroke, a physician was faced with choices: could he or she make the right ones on the basis of the NINDS stroke trial? Furlan was skeptical.

Zivin brought up another issue in the same domain—ethics. He asserted it was no longer acceptable to enroll stroke patients in placebo-controlled trials if they reached the hospital within 3 hours. Those patients should be given tPA. To let them be treated with either nothing or with another thrombolytic was actually to cross an ethical divide. He was being purposely provocative. Zivin knew very well that trials using streptokinase were proceeding in Australia, Italy, and elsewhere in Europe. With tPA, the European Cooperative Acute Stroke Study had already published its negative results with a longer time window, so a further incarnation was being planned.

The upshot was that, at the final session after a long weekend, a roundtable discussion of international experts provided a forum for confusion. The issue Zivin had raised became a flashpoint. One of the renowned moderators put the question to the distinguished group before the elite audience: was it ethical to continue running placebo-controlled trials for stroke patients who present within 3 hours?

As 10 participants weighed in, most said: Yes, it is ethical.

Then came a question from the audience. A woman stood up to identify herself as a local neurologist, responsible for the sector of Copenhagen where the conference was taking place.

"If any of you have a stroke tonight, I will be taking care of you. And if you come in with a stroke, do you want me to give you tPA?"

Now the roundtable turned on a dime: all but two said they wanted tPA. The meeting broke up with boos and laughter. It was a foretaste of what was to come.

One roundtable participant, Louis R. Caplan, was perhaps the best-known stroke expert in the United States if not the world. Indeed, he was a father of contemporary stroke neurology, one of the successors to C. Miller Fisher and Raymond D. Adams, who were acknowledged progenitors of the field. A prominent authority and Harvard professor, Caplan was author of a lucidly written textbook; his opinions were widely followed and respected. When he weighed in on tPA, as he did in a 1997 "debate" in the *New England Journal of Medicine*, he helped intensify hostility and polarize opinion. He was the chief author of "Thrombolysis—Not a Panacea for Ischemic Stroke," a piece also signed by three highly respected colleagues: Jay P. Mohr of Columbia University and, from Harvard Medical School, J. Philip Kistler and Walter Koroshetz. Together they were a powerful voice in American neurology. Their evaluation of tPA set in motion a negative juggernaut that would eventually stall and turn back of its own accord—and their own minds would change—but not before having provoked considerable negative repercussions.

From a rhetorical point of view, the 1997 "debate" did not rely on subtlety from either side. Caplan and his colleagues presented the case against tPA while Jim Grotta, for the NINDS study investigators, wrote the terse response.

Caplan and colleagues objected to the NINDS study finding that tPA should be used to treat all ischemic strokes regardless of subtype. "We think," they wrote, "that patients are better served by accurate diagnosis and appropriate specific therapy than by a shotgun approach." He and his co-authors criticized the American Heart Association and American Academy of Neurology for endorsing the treatment so quickly upon FDA approval: "Rather than accept any delay, [these organizations] choose not to require or even suggest tests to define the causative pathophysiology and detect underlying occlusive vascular lesions."

In addition, stroke had never before been seen in terms of fast treatment, and Caplan and others did not like it now. They doubted the full significance of the 3-hour time-to-treatment window. "Although time is important, so is the specificity of the diagnosis," they insisted, adding, "No one would choose to give an effective but potentially dangerous drug to patients who do not have the target problem that the drug treats." They pointed to potential misdiagnoses and to new imaging procedures, such as magnetic resonance imaging (MRI), that might affect treatment. Some strokes might turn out to be better treated by injecting tPA directly into the occluded artery rather than intravenously—though there was no evidence for this. Caplan and co-authors ended with an appeal for further investigation and argued for the use of tPA only when "occlusive lesions" were demonstrably present. They raised the danger that, if administered to "all patients with ischemic stroke," the drug would foreclose on needed research.

Responding, Jim Grotta brusquely noted the obvious—that the 3-hour window was developed in consequence of both animal studies and clinical experience; that tPA benefitted all subtypes of ischemic stroke; and that the drug did not increase mortality, "early or late." Forty-eight percent of tPA-treated patients but just 36% of placebo patients would return home instead of being sent to a nursing home or rehabilitation center. Diagnostic errors for treated patients in the NINDS study had proved not to be above 1%. Grotta disputed the notion that using tPA as standard treatment would halt further research. "Nor should such academic concerns," he wrote, and one senses clenched teeth, "retard the use of an effective therapy for patients, in any case."

Indeed, Jim Grotta was not happy with the whole debate. Much as he liked and remained friends with Lou Caplan and the other participants, the experience left a residue of bitterness. He had simply offered to write a review article for the *New England Journal of Medicine* and instead was roped into an argument he thought unnecessary. At first he had refused: "I didn't really think debate was appropriate, because the results of the NINDS trial were positive and there weren't any studies like the NINDS trial that were negative." At last he agreed, but, as he feared, the "Boston neurologists" weighed in with their unenthusiastic views. He recalled: "That just put such a bad taste in my mouth. Here we had a treatment and rather than embracing it and trying to get people to treat stroke, we had the stroke experts who were trying to throw arrows at the data."

The debate was not innocuous, thought Grotta. Together with Genentech's anemic marketing, the drug lost momentum. For himself, Grotta turned away from efforts to proselytize or defend. At the University of Texas Medical School at Houston, where he directed the stroke program, he demonstrated what thrombolysis could do. By 2009 Grotta would be able to claim that some 60% of patients who managed to reach 911 would be rushed to a stroke center within 2 hours, and 20% of these emergency cases would be treated with tPA. Those numbers did not reach the level that might come with greater public education, but they were significant. "We probably use more tPA than anyplace in the world and treat more people with tPA than anybody, and we publish the results." He did not become a doctor to sell a treatment. "I mean, if people don't want to use it, screw them. It's too bad because the patients are the ones that suffer. But my job isn't to go out there and convince Dr. Joe Jones to use a drug if he doesn't want to use it. But I'm going to use it and teach people to use it."

Others tacked sails in the same direction. At San Diego, Pat Lyden created a training course. Genentech had stopped advertising tPA for stroke but would pay for this. Several weekends a year about 30 doctors—neurologists, emergency physicians, internists—would show up. "We promised that if you came on a Friday morning, when you left Saturday afternoon you would be able to push tPA by yourself." He created a syllabus that included editorials by skeptics like Lou Caplan. They'd go over the data and then discuss hypothetical cases. "Stroke Camp," as he called it, was successful. "And in fact, on at least two occasions doctors went home and on Sunday after Stroke Camp they treated patients."

But it was a drop in the bucket. Similar efforts were sponsored by the American Heart Association and other organizations. Studies consistently showed that community hospitals could provide tPA according to protocol, that concerns over doctors failing if they were not academic experts were misplaced. One intriguing result, published in 2001, was that a patient was significantly more likely to receive tPA if he or she had a stroke in the western half of the United States than in the east. Perhaps there was something to the view that the hostile reception from Boston neurologists carried a lasting impact.

With any treatment there is an expected learning curve, and with tPA there was recognition that growing awareness would take time. Zivin, in conversations with the Genentech researchers, made it clear that a good guess was 10 years, based on what had happened with heart attack, for knowledge about the drug to filter into awareness. For stroke, there were personnel to train, equipment to buy, and protocol to develop that were suited to individual emergency rooms. In separate 1997 articles, Joe Broderick, one of the key members of the team at the University of Cincinnati, and Barbara Tilley outlined concrete examples. Expectations ran high at first.

The NINDS study investigators held out high expectations that neurologists would lead the way. Brain specialists above all, they thought, would understand the promise of tPA. They would advise at-risk patients, work with hospital emergency physicians, give tPA, and teach others to use it. Undoubtedly it would take time before wide advocacy of the drug took hold and the urgent character of stroke penetrated doctor and patient awareness. Because most stroke victims are elderly, Medicare would need to provide appropriate reimbursement; private insurance companies would follow suit. The experience of the cardiologists constituted a precedent. A decade earlier, during the 1980s, they enthusiastically sought tPA. Indeed, around the time the drug was approved in 1987, they were "salivating" for it. Soon after, emergency physicians too were clamoring to use it. For stroke, would not neurologists similarly lead the way?

They would not. "Neurologists," said Pat Lyden, "just couldn't be bothered."

"So all these guys," recalled Steve Horowitz, "were sitting in their offices and had very pleasant jobs because there was very little night call or ER call and stuff like that. They were loath to get up in the middle of the night or disturb their medical practices in their offices in order to run down to a hospital to evaluate a patient for tPA."

As the NINDS study investigators came grimly to view matters, the hostile, thumbs-down reception that neurologists accorded tPA for stroke was due not to the drug or issues of efficacy; rather, it was due to the make-up of the specialty itself and the people in it.

In general, when physicians specialize they choose disciplines that suit them personally. Neurology attracted brainy but not hands-on kinds of people. The profession valued observation rather than intervention. Most neurology practices were office-based; seldom did neurologists deal with emergencies. If tPA was more like a surgical procedure than a drug treatment, neurologists were far from being surgeons. Much of their time was devoted to diagnosing and treating illnesses such as Parkinson's disease, Alzheimer's disease, and multiple sclerosis. They dealt mainly in slow diseases, not fast diseases.

"We think of ourselves, or used to, as cognitive people," said Horowitz. "We would localize a process in the nervous system; we would spend inordinate amounts of time making a diagnosis. It was thought to be a very erudite specialty." With irony, to boot: "And after you finally arrived at a diagnosis, you couldn't do anything for the various diseases."

For stroke, neurologists were seldom first responders. "The clinical responsibility for diagnosis and treatment (what little were available) was the responsibility primarily of family physicians and internists," remembered Murray Goldstein, a former NINDS director and U.S. Assistant Surgeon General. "[N]eurologists and neurosurgeons typically were involved as consultants in unusual or difficult cases." Mostly, they consulted on rehabilitation after a stroke was complete. Whether it was 1936 or 1996, neurologists did not see themselves rushing to the hospital to evaluate patients, many of whom would be ineligible for tPA, anyway.

Horowitz, the gruff-spoken New York neurologist—and local principal investigator for the NINDS trial at Long Island Jewish Medical Center—was an exception. He helped write the original NINDS paper for the *New England Journal of Medicine* and in 1998 published in the *Archives of Neurology* the most down-to-earth recognition that the drug was meeting stiff resistance. Its title told it all: "Neurologists, Get Off Your Hands!"

Like the other NINDS study investigators, Horowitz had been talking about tPA to neurologists at gatherings across the country. He was writing now, he said, "to convey my impressions of the lack of enthusiasm for this therapy exhibited by neurologists at places where I have spoken." He encountered skepticism and denial, not enthusiasm in "discussions [that] centered around why t-PA cannot or should not be used, rather than how it could be used."

Horowitz was perhaps the first, in print anyhow, to implicate the neurological tradition: "My personal belief is that modern neurology bears the legacy of the specialty when it was more philosophical, intellectual, and phenomenological in nature, more notable for cogitation than action." He found "substantial resistance among many neurologists to do anything more than debate, or consider, often at arm's length, any possibility of using t-PA…" He acknowledged practical issues: compensation and disruption to office practice. But continuing negativism "forecloses on the immediate opportunity to treat a common disorder having significant morbidity and mortality on its own, and for which no other agent is currently available."

In one respect Horowitz proved mistaken: "Emergency medicine physicians and internists, and possibly generalists, will surely use t-PA if we do not, certainly to the detriment of our specialty and, most likely, to the patient as well." As it turned out, if neurologists were not to lead, other doctors would not follow.

Neurologists protested both privately and publicly, although in different and telling ways. Like Steve Horowitz, NINDS study investigator Jim Grotta got an earful when he gave talks: "I don't know how many neurologists came up to me and were very upset at me for publishing and giving lectures about tPA because they said it was going to change their lives. They were now going to have to be on call to the emergency room and be basically emergency responders, whereas neurologists had never had to do that before." To a point he could understand their reluctance: emergency work was not what they signed up for. "But that's not a reason" said Grotta, "to trash the study."

In print, though, the issue was invariably safety. A prominent example was "Tissue-Type Plasminogen Activator Should Not Be Used in Acute Ischemic Stroke," published as part of yet another debate in the *Archives of Neurology* and reprinted in *Archives of Family Medicine* in early 1997. Neurologist Jack E. Riggs underscored the danger of harm. (As far as Horowitz was concerned, the article offered only "a pedantic discussion of the psychology of how patients give consent.") Riggs acknowledged the results: some 31% of patients showed an excellent outcome at 3 months, and this represented a 50% improvement over doing nothing. But he accused the NINDS study investigators of minimizing the "risk of early iatrogenic [doctor-induced] death." He asked: "Would you risk a 12% chance of an improved neurological outcome at 3 months following ischemic stroke against a 3% chance of early death from rt-PA-induced intracerebral hemorrhage?"

By "early death" Riggs could only, by inference, be suggesting that more tPA patients died soon after their stroke than placebo patients; by 3 months, mortality for both groups was statistically the same. Framing the issue in this way created a wedge that seemed to reveal iatrogenic harm: a patient who did not die the day of the stroke but within a few weeks. Riggs was mistaken, however: as was already clear from the 1995 paper, the original data showed no spike in the rate of early death from tPA.

Cognitive dissonance, a durable concept in social psychology, addresses the fact that people want to be consistent in their thoughts and actions. So when an individual experiences two cognitive elements in conflict, he or she will feel pressure to reduce or eliminate the associated and unpleasant sensations. Rationalization may be used—for example, "I only smoke one pack of cigarettes a day"—but when the magnitude of dissonance is great, simple reasoning fails. This was the case with tPA for stroke. Although neurologists had never treated stroke as an emergency, that was not a good professional reason not to start now; it was an excuse. The clinical trials with the other major thrombolytic drug, streptokinase, had failed, but you could not get away from the successful NINDS trials or the fact that tPA was an endogenous substance with greater specificity. Clearly it would be unacceptable for neurologists to argue, individually or as a group, that they would not treat with tPA because it involved getting up in the middle of the night or being poorly compensated.

But recourse to authority and the issue of toxicity represented a different type of solution. Such articles as Riggs's and the "debate" in the *New England Journal of Medicine* helped neurologists, individually and as a group, to justify continued resolve not to use tPA. If Lou Caplan, one of the fathers of stroke neurology, questioned it, his authority stood for something. If Jack Riggs brought up the ethical issue of iatrogenic harm, the discomfort associated with not treating stroke could indeed be made to disappear.

But to test rationalization and cognitive dissonance, put them to the side for a moment and ask: What was the real risk of cerebral hemorrhage? Concern about a relationship between thrombolytic drugs and bleeding strokes was not new. In general, hemorrhagic stroke was more closely associated with a catastrophic outcome than ischemic stroke, and the transformation of an ischemic into a bleeding stroke was, on the face of it, highly undesirable. Thrombolysis for whatever indication with streptokinase, according to the 1980 NIH consensus, carried serious risks of cerebral hemorrhage. The original package insert itself for tPA, when it was approved for heart attack, stated that it was contraindicated for stroke; only after the NINDS trial was it changed. The larger story, however, was at once simpler and more complicated.

We have stressed elsewhere in this book (see especially Chapter 2) how incomplete knowledge about clot formation and clot dissolution has in the past provoked scientific investigation but also generated unsupported speculation about what actually happens within the cerebrovascular system during a stroke. The problem of tPA in connection with hemorrhage turns out to be another instance. Despite solid knowledge derived from all aspects of hemodynamics and pathophysiology, a complete account of brain hemorrhage has proved elusive, and so it gave rise to an incomplete picture that, once again, proved ripe for misinterpretation. The fact was that, with respect to tPA, neurologists were apt to react with far greater concern about hemorrhage than was warranted; one might even call it hysteria.

Zivin had investigated cerebral hemorrhage after publication of his 1985 paper on the rabbit model for tPA because, as Genentech developed the drug for use with heart attack in the 1980s, a bleeding stroke was the most serious potential complication. At one point, he was brought to the company's South San Francisco headquarters and questioned in front of a large audience of Genentech researchers. David Botstein, vice president in charge of science, asked him directly about the cause or causes of cerebral hemorrhage. Although it did not feel good to give an unsatisfactory answer in front of about 75 scientists, he had to say he did not know. "Our current understanding of hemorrhagic transformation," as he would put it later in an article he wrote with Pat Lyden, "lacks empirical and theoretical support and detail." He went on to conduct experiments—with some support from Genentech—that would demonstrate that hemorrhagic conversion in stroked rabbits was significantly more likely to occur with streptokinase than with tPA. Genentech scientists had taken note of this work, and their support had encouraged the company to provide the drug for the NINDS study.

Not to say there were no theories, of course. A number of possible causes of hemorrhage had been demonstrated, together with classification by type and location. But the actual train of events that caused blood to leak into the brain remained a description in hypothetical terms. This was true in 1989 and remains so today. What may be said with confidence is that this incomplete understanding affected the reception that neurologists accorded tPA.

Essentially, stroke-related hemorrhages are of two kinds. The most serious, known as *parenchymatous hemorrhage*, involves the rupture of a blood vessel and bleeding into the brain. (The term *parenchyma* is a general one that refers to the functional substance of an organ.) Such strokes are typically catastrophic and often fatal. A good example is probably President Franklin Delano Roosevelt's almost instantaneous death from a massive hemorrhagic stroke.

But other bleeding strokes start out ischemic; these are known as *hemorrhagic transformations*. How they actually evolve and the gravity of such a turn of events are based on a set of individual and unknown factors. There does exist a long-dominant theory—still in wide circulation today. In 1951 C. Miller Fisher and Raymond D. Adams, who became the most celebrated stroke authorities for a whole generation and more, published a brief paper on a series of autopsies of patients who had suffered from cerebrovascular disease. Based on the size and location of damaged tissue and embolisms, if any could be found, they theorized that hemorrhagic transformation would occur after a clot spontaneously dissolved. The idea was simple. A clot in a major artery would starve small vessels downstream and engender structural damage. When the clot dissolved, wholly or partially, the return of blood and repressurization of those formerly occluded vessels could cause what was sometimes called a "blowout"—much as can happen when a defective bicycle tire is pumped back full of air. Although neurologists in principle recognized that the "clot lysis/distal migration theory," as it was called, might be incomplete, its simplicity made it attractive as a general explanation of how an ischemic stroke might be transformed into a bleeding stroke.

Genentech scientists, when they learned that fundamental uncertainty plagued the theory, did something that would be unknown in a purely academic environment: they provided Zivin with support in efforts to develop an animal model of hemorrhagic transformation. From 1987 to 1991 Zivin and Pat Lyden ran several hundred studies in individual rabbits in which a blood clot was introduced into the major cerebral artery. The principal finding was that with or without thrombolysis with tPA, hemorrhage could be found in some 30% of animals. That represented a base rate. In addition, they showed that both aspirin and streptokinase were associated with more hemorrhages, whereas that was not the case with the anticoagulant heparin.

These results cast doubt on the "blowout" model of transformational hemorrhage. In addition, reviewing the literature, Zivin confirmed earlier research suggesting that leakage through surrounding capillaries could account for the blood found around infarcts after an ischemic stroke—not invariably rupture of vessel walls. Further, he pointed to recent studies in people that showed hemorrhagic transformation was common—in one set of data, occurring in from 15% to 43% of untreated strokes. In short, some bleeding in the case of ischemic stroke was not even necessarily dangerous. It remained true that for clot dissolution with thrombolytic therapy, timing was important for saving the brain, but "transformation is of little concern if the patient enjoys a simultaneous clinical improvement."

Nothing related to these clarifications concerning hemorrhagic transformation found its way into the NINDS study, which was completing the first of its two trials when the article was published in 1993. Overweening concern about hemorrhage was thus a legacy burden, as it were, of previous studies combined with received wisdom. In retrospect, the study's protocol provided an overly conservative definition of "symptomatic hemorrhage." Patients who after treatment showed cognitive or physical deterioration of any kind would undergo a CT scan. Any image that indicated bleeding, no matter how trivial and regardless of behavioral recovery, was taken to be symptomatic hemorrhagic transformation due to tPA—whether this was the case or not. The NINDS study investigators scrupulously reported every instance discovered within 36 hours of treatment. Mike Welch recalls, "We were very, very, very concerned" about hemorrhage and, he added, so was the FDA. He communicated with agency officials after looking closely at the details of each reported hemorrhage.

The result was an exaggerated assessment of risk. At the end of the NINDS trials came the famous numbers: 6% more hemorrhages with tPA, half of which were fatal. Yet the drug clearly worked and the FDA approved its use in stroke because 3-month mortality and morbidity were at parity whether a patient received tPA or a placebo, hemorrhage or not.

Taken out of original context, if numbers from the NINDS study implied tPA would cause the death of 3 patients in 100, the risk was exaggerated (this is explained more fully in Chapter 10). Just note for the moment that concern became viral in the literature; it was everywhere cited and often misinterpreted for a wider public. So it has continued over the years. In a popular health care book entitled *Worried Sick*, for example, Nortin M. Hadler, a rheumatologist and critic of overmedication, included a strikingly misinformed paragraph about tPA for stroke, warning of "the 6 percent in whom the infusion [of tPA] causes far more catastrophic bleeding into the brain than nearly all strokes." In the hope his stroke would be a transient ischemic attack, he adds, "I'll take my chances with the natural history." Examples of such thinking, hampered by insufficient information and confusion over statistics, could be multiplied by the dozens.

Disputes over tPA for stroke were by no means confined to a couple of debates, articles in journals, or letters to the editor. Among neurologists, conflict raged and simmered and spurted forth time and again over the course of about 8 years.

"No issue has caused greater controversy than the view that intravenous tPA should be a standard form of therapy for acute stroke," wrote Australian neurologists Geoffrey A. Donnan and Stephen M. Davis in 2003. They had concluded in 2001 that "Enough is Enough!" and advised the field to acknowledge the drug worked as indicated and to move on to randomized trials testing it beyond the 3-hour time window. But the same year, a British physician, Richard Iain Lindley, argued for further trials within that timeframe, writing that the NINDS trial was "unusually positive and in general, has, been overemphasized." He asked: "Were they simply lucky?" Pat Lyden replied that the original study and subsequent trials "have been digested, criticized, confirmed, supplemented with additional data and diffused widely." And so it went.

In a sense, tPA made progress. It advanced in the minds of neurologists, strokologists, and academics who were at first skeptical. The drug, they now began to acknowledge, was effective. These were the people most likely to be informed about the clutch of trials that tested tPA with longer times-to-treatment and in various community settings. New results and retrospective studies only bore out the original results None broke new ground so much as softened resistance and over time created new advocates.

Most trials to test tPA, conducted both in the United States and internationally, were in effect confirmatory of the NINDS study. For a long time none was a global success, but all were revealing in their failures and validated the short time-to-treatment window. Thus, the European Cooperative Acute Stroke Study (ECASS) had a 6-hour clock and, though it failed to show benefit within that timeframe, patients treated within 3 hours improved more than both controls and patients treated between 3 to 6 hours. The Alteplase Thrombolysis for Acute Noninterventional Therapy in Ischemic Stroke (ATLANTIS) study similarly succeeded when results were analyzed for tPA-treated patients within 3 hours. Eventually, data from the NINDS, ECASS, and ATLANTIS trials were pooled and showed the same highly significant favorable outcome at 3 months; results also hinted that the time window might be extended to 4.5 hours.

The NINDS study investigators also mined their own trial for further publications. In 1999 the NINDS Stroke Study Group published follow-up results which showed that patients maintained the magnitude of benefit at 6 and 12 months after treatment. Those who received tPA continued to live and function significantly better than patients who received placebo. There was still no overall difference in mortality—an important fact, which again suggested that patients for whom a stroke was fatal tended to suffer a massive event that would end their lives whether it remained ischemic or turned into a bleeding stroke.

Finally, it also became clear that tPA for stroke need not be confined to academic medical centers: community hospitals could administer tPA if they tried. A couple of years after the NINDS results were published, a so-called phase IV trial assessed 389 patients from 57 medical centers in the United States; the results showed the drug could be safely used outside the strict environment of the randomized control trial in an academic medical center. One study, out of the Cleveland hospital system, counted an excess of protocol violations and brought about an adverse result, but it was to remain a lone outlier. In 1999 the Cleveland group undertook a quality improvement program and 4 years later published a paper showing outcomes similar to the NINDS study.

Over time and with advancing success in the wake of the NINDS study, neurologists could not sustain feeling good about not advocating the use of tPA. One by one the leaders in the field, and afterwards many of the rank and file, changed their minds.

Jack Riggs, for example, subsequently came to an accommodation with tPA. At West Virginia University Healthcare, where he still works, he said in 2009:

"We use tPA all the time." He would still cite the obsolete extrapolation that a doctor will on average treat eight patients with tPA before he benefits one. (In fact, subsequently this figure was recalculated—we will explain why and how in Chapter 10—to reveal that tPA benefits at least one patient in three.) Although surprised and impressed by the way the drug can be safely used in community hospitals, he still does not like tPA much and says: "I'm still not overly impressed with its utility." And while acknowledging that the drug has probably started to enhance awareness of stroke, he remains pessimistic: "The number of people treated with tPA is really tiny." Which, of course, is true.

It took a couple of years, but Lou Caplan himself changed his mind—at least, on the big issue as to whether tPA worked and should be used. He still believed the drug had been approved and endorsed prematurely, but he was nothing if not forthright in his about-face. "Approval of tPA was a wake-up call," he wrote. "*Stroke can and should be treated* [emphasis in original]." He would eventually encourage the use of webcam-based telemedicine by which treating physicians of any stripe could consult with neurologists. "Stroke patients must be hustled quickly into medical centers, and doctors and hospitals must become prepared and able to treat them." However, with signature idiosyncrasy, Caplan still recommended withholding tPA from patients when symptoms suggested the "lacunar syndrome"—occlusions in the cerebral arterioles (the smallest of the arteries) often undetectable by imaging. (The original NINDS study suggested otherwise.) And he very much remained Lou Caplan in arguing for nuanced diagnosis and use of advanced imaging wherever possible. To give tPA just by the CT scan and the clock "doesn't make any sense to me."

Other highly regarded stroke doctors also changed their minds about tPA toward the beginning of the millennium. This included the trio of leading physicians—Kistler, Koroshetz, and Mohr—who had signed Lou Caplan's "no panacea" article in the *New England Journal of Medicine*. "Steadily accumulating data continue to justify current guidelines for use of tPA in stroke," wrote Mohr in an editorial in *JAMA* in 2000, "and demonstrate that low complication rates can be achieved with proper use of this therapy." Another early skeptic, Anthony Furlan of the Cleveland Clinic, soon enough admitted to be puzzled by the reluctance of doctors to use tPA. "Looking back," he said, "I now find it curious that many physicians were willing to use treatments like coumadin or heparin when there were no efficacy data, yet many now will not use intravenous tissue plasminogen activator (tPA) when there are efficacy data." He became a strong advocate and joined a list that grew longer and ultimately, among stroke doctors, morphed into consensus.

In sum, to convince neurologists to treat stroke patients with tPA proved neither simple nor easy, but it did start to happen. "It might be easier," quipped

Mike Welch around 1996, "to get a neurologist into bed than out of bed." By 2002 that situation was at least, if not rectified, a reverse work-in-progress.

But neurologists not only were familiar with stroke symptoms as specialists; they represented potential leaders to gain acceptance for tPA within the larger medical community. All doctors who provided primary care for adult patients could learn to use tPA with stroke, much as they acquired the skills of emergency intervention in heart attack. The fairly simple set of intellectual tools could be taught in medical school or learned by older doctors as short courses in continuing medical education. With this larger context in mind, the alleviation of reticence and skepticism on the part of neurologists represented a welcome advance.

But by the time consensus among neurologists started to coalesce, shortly after the turn of the century, about 2002, tPA for stroke faced resistance from another group. Emergency physicians, unlike neurologists, were first responders. They did have a responsibility to treat stroke—and with tPA a new and unprecedented opportunity. But the antagonism of a large number, sponsored by the leadership of their professional organizations, was particularly severe. It was slow to diminish, rages still in some quarters, and represents—as is discussed in the next chapter—a lost connection between science and medicine.

What Emergency? | 6

*I*t is hard to overstate how powerfully the NINDS study investigators came to dislike everything that Jerome Hoffman, an avatar in emergency medicine, wrote and said about tPA for stroke. Steve Horowitz, for one, declined to recall his name, citing with bluff scorn "some guy from California." John Marler dismissed Hoffman as a skilled debater who "relies little on fact." Others hinted darkly at the ultimate verdict of history. About this doctor, who came to represent and embody resistance to tPA for stroke, some colleagues declined to talk on the record. Others pointed to the irony that the physician who campaigned so prominently against tPA works and teaches at an institution where it is used all the time. Not only did stroke neurologists resent what Jerry Hoffman was doing; he eventually generated frustration, antagonism, and even embarrassment in his own field.

More than one NINDS study investigator suggested that any account of stroke and tPA should studiously ignore Jerome Hoffman and not cite him, at least by name. But he was highly visible and helped to foment distrust of the drug on an international scale. All agreed he was intelligent, charismatic, and influential. The story he generated would be entertaining if it were not tragic. For, if emergency room physicians had decided to use tPA for stroke with the same zeal as they earlier employed with heart attack, it might well have meant faster acceptance, training of everybody involved, and changing the rules by which acute stroke patients were treated. Given the crucial importance of public education, it probably still would have taken 10 years or more before the message brought substantial numbers to the emergency room fast. Yet it would have happened sooner and without the corrosive conflict that persists to this day.

But it must be emphasized that Hoffman's leverage was packaged by context and circumstance. Emergency physicians' skepticism, reticence, and fear of the treating the brain with tPA were due first of all to the neurologists, and that original sticking-point should not be underplayed. Emergency doctors had been positive on clot-busting with heart attack because cardiologists were proactive in promoting tPA when it was first used in the 1980s. "They were all over it," recalls Bill Barsan, one of the earliest academic emergency physicians. "They [the cardiologists] expected us to do our part in that algorithm when the heart attack patients hit the door. And they set it up from the beginning as very much a team effort. And that didn't happen with stroke care."

Indeed, collaboration forms a crucial aspect, almost a way of life, for emergency physicians. They work with other specialists, not only cardiologists for heart attack but trauma surgeons, toxicologists, neurosurgeons, and radiologists of every stripe. Neurologists, by contrast with all such specialists, did not show up. As we have seen, they made it clear in the late 1990s, so far as stroke was concerned, they were not interested in being on call or treating stroke as an emergency.

"A lot of ER docs thought they were being hung out to dry," says Barsan. "The backlash from the field came when nobody was creating a collaboration and the default person was the emergency doctor. So if a person didn't get a thrombolytic for an acute stroke, it was their fault."

What were emergency physicians to do? Their hospital pharmacies stocked the drug they used for heart attack that now, in addition, carried an indication for stroke. Without support from neurologists or, in the vast majority of cases, from hospital administrators, they were confronted with a choice. Emergency physicians could become advocates of a revolutionary treatment for stroke—or maybe not.

When Jerry Hoffman, one of their leaders, came down hard on the drug and the NINDS study, he found among these doctors a large and receptive audience, many enthusiastic in their rejection of tPA for stroke and hopeful of finding a good reason why.

Emergency medicine is a recent specialty, scarcely half a century old. It grew up centered around the hospital rather than an academic environment and was not formally organized until the late 1960s; only in 1989 did it become a primary board-certified specialty. "It was bred by new social and political conditions, borne out of service needs, and nurtured by a few maverick physicians," writes Brian J. Zink in *Anyone, Anything, Anytime: A History of Emergency Medicine*. "It developed as an outsider looking in—a populist favorite shunned by the medical establishment." But it grew rapidly, and just 10 years after the American College of Emergency Physicians (ACEP) was founded in 1968, some 30 universities offered residency training programs. Today the popular specialty has about 25,000 members.

Although not among its Midwestern pioneers, Jerome Hoffman nicely fit the idiosyncratic niche that emergency medicine came to occupy. He belonged to its first generation, a Princeton graduate who as a young man protested the Vietnam War, studied theatrical literature at Columbia University, and wanted to be a writer before turning to medicine. He settled for becoming a professor of clinical and emergency medicine at UCLA. There he became "a force in emergency medicine in the old-fashioned way," according to an admiring article: "by going against the grain."

During the 1980s Hoffman became exceptionally well known in the field after he and another physician, Richard Bukata, developed a popular series of audiotapes for continuing medical education. As to be expected in a field that interacts with so many specialties and treats such a wide range of disorders, keeping up with new developments is of special importance for emergency medicine. Bukata and Hoffman provided emergency physicians with a much needed, widely subscribed-to service. Repartee between practical-minded Bukata and Hoffman, the erudite academic, was both instructive and entertaining. The pair, writes Brian Zink, "played a big role in setting the national tone for emergency medicine in their reactions [to] and analysis [of] new studies, drugs, and practice methods."

Hoffman considered himself a skeptic and made clinical epidemiology his area of expertise. He participated in original research, but his major role was as critic. He was a self-described gadfly and "odd man out." He had a biting sense of humor. Once he and a colleague wrote a scathingly sarcastic letter to a medical journal criticizing a brief report on "high altitude flatus expulsion"—a rare enough disorder, to be sure. "[T]he importance of the syndrome cannot be overstated" wrote Hoffman tongue-in-cheek. He urged creation of SCHTOOOL— the "Society (for the) Collection and Historical Tabulation of Olfactory and Otherwise malOdorous Literature."

Global mistrust of the pharmaceutical industry was another arrow in Hoffman's critical quiver. To salutary concerns over the moral rectitude of physicians and seductive claims of drug companies, he brought an absolutist approach. He was an early critic of the multiple ways by which big pharmaceutical companies insinuate themselves into medical education, and how they design and market products with an overriding yet unstated focus on profit.

Together with an acolyte, science writer Jeanne Lenzer, Hoffman was one of the main talking heads in a health care documentary entitled *Money Talks*. Hoffman himself was unwilling to accept even a ballpoint pen with a company logo; it compromised integrity.

An additional crucial but overlooked component to Hoffman's view of medicine was a considerable degree of therapeutic pessimism, whether fully acknowledged or not. Recalling his own youthful enthusiasm for medicine, he wrote of his more mature understanding that physicians "rarely save (really save) even a single life." If only he had known, he wrote, "[t]hat it is almost impossible to be competent, no less masterful, given the complexity of what we do. That we routinely fail despite our best efforts. That almost all our decisions are shrouded in uncertainty."

Although he would insist that his work was driven by the data he analyzed, Hoffman's distrust of pharmaceutical companies, his exclusive focus on epidemiology, and his cultivated pessimism all appear to have helped, in a synergistic way, to shape his evaluation of tPA for stroke.

Upfront it must be emphasized that emergency physicians never spoke with a single voice about stroke and tPA. When Bill Barsan graduated from medical school in the mid-1970s, he already planned on an academic career, still rare in emergency medicine. The tPA pilot studies in the late 1980s provided a research opportunity. NINDS administrator John Marler buttonholed him at a conference in New Orleans. "Tell me realistically," Barsan recalls Marler asking, "if a patient hits the door with a stroke, what's the soonest you could get somebody treated—a CT scan, consent, and drug in?" Marler was acting at the behest of his boss, Mike Walker, who wanted unvarnished input from the emergency room. What was the shortest time to treatment, according to an ER doctor?

Barsan thought about it and replied: "An hour." His reply confirmed what Marler thought, that some strokes could be treated within about 90 minutes overall: an hour for the patient to reach the emergency department and be prepared to receive tPA, plus half an hour for the drug to begin to work.

Barsan went on to work with Tom Brott in Cincinnati and, in fact, he injected the first patient with tPA in the first small, open-label trial. The patient, who had lost speech and was completely paralyzed on the right side of his body, had an on-the-table response, improving within minutes.

Emergency doctors won recognition during the NINDS trials as key players in providing the treatment. For the larger study, Marler and Walker insisted that each participating hospital include an emergency physician as a co-investigator. At the time this was an unusual step. "It used to be," Barsan recalls, "that if a neurologist or pulmonary doctor or a cardiologist, or anybody else basically, wanted to do studies that involved emergency patients, usually what they'd do is they would write up their protocol and they'd get it approved, and they'd get their funding, and then they'd come down to the emergency room and say, 'Oh, by the way, we're doing a study on your patients.'"

But for most neurologists, interaction with the emergency room prior to the NINDS study was far from an everyday occurrence. If few emergency physicians had gone through a neurology rotation during medical school, most neurologists were happy to forget their student turn in the ER. Although an emergency doctor could readily learn to recognize and diagnose stroke—in spite of later claims to the contrary—signs and symptoms are more variable than those with heart attack. The problems of training and expertise could be met, but they were real.

"There is no diagnostic dilemma," dryly points out Phillip A. Scott, a colleague of Barsan's, "when a patient comes in with a .44 Glock hole in his chest." Simple diagnosis was the nature of much emergency medicine, at least when it came to proactive treatment. With heart attack, too, the therapeutic window is generally longer and the outcome clear-cut: the patient lives to walk away or grows worse and dies. But of prime importance, stroke often cripples when it is not lethal. The final outcome, weeks and months later, not only varies greatly but essentially cannot be forecast. For emergency physicians in academic settings, the solution to all such issues—including hostility and indifference on the part of neurologists—was to establish an acute stroke protocol, the "rules of the game."

By the time the NINDS study ended, Bill Barsan was working with the Brain Injury Group at the University of Michigan. After learning of the results, he immediately prepared to use tPA. He brought in Phil Scott, who also had been an emergency resident in Cincinnati and was familiar with the NINDS study. In early 1996 Barsan and Scott put into operation a system to evaluate stroke patients. They operated autonomously. At first, there were no stroke neurologists with the Brain Injury Group.

"Basically we were the people on point call," said Barsan. "When the call came in, we were the ones who responded. We would make the decision as to who got tPA and who didn't."

The 23-page protocol, for all it might sound daunting, could be quickly completed with the aid of a nurse and radiologist. If a person could follow a checklist, he or she could safely decide whether to give tPA. The Brain Injury Group was using the drug "off-label"—an accepted albeit sometimes legally risky choice—even before the FDA approved the indication for stroke.

Organized adoption of tPA for stroke was not typical, however. Other emergency teams appeared, most at research-oriented, university-based institutions and often in some way associated with the NINDS study. These early adopters constituted the nub of a wider movement toward certified stroke centers— hospitals designated as the ones to which stroke victims should be preferentially transported. By the late 1990s, too, some hospitals put into place a "stroke protocol" that included use of tPA but did not necessarily involve comprehensive training of all staff. This situation put the emergency physician at the center of a decision-making process, often without the full support of a neurologist, around a disorder for which custom and practice had long dictated that, beyond stabilizing the patient, nothing could be done. As one consequence, more than 4,000 hospitals in the United States became environments in which antagonism of emergency physicians toward tPA could be encouraged and cultivated.

When time came for Jerome Hoffman to evaluate the NINDS study, he chose to underplay and devalue its principal positive finding, the absolute benefit of 11% to 13% for treatment with tPA. Rather, he characterized the overall benefit as modest because, due to the narrow time window, only a small percentage of stroke patients would be judged eligible to receive the drug. That led him to suggest that thrombolysis "could only help, at most, 1 of every 125 patients." This observation may have been true at the time but ignored the obvious: acute stroke care could be vastly improved in terms of time-to-treatment.

While acknowledging the study was methodologically sound, Hoffman brought up the much-noted imbalances between the tPA and placebo groups. He declared, as others had done before him, that the positive results of the entire study might thus be due to chance. In what would become a standard argument among the dedicated naysayers, he wrote that "the benefit [in the NINDS study] was primarily in patients treated less than 90 minutes after symptom onset." As a consequence, Hoffman made much of his doubts that tPA could be used effectively outside the academic medical centers where the NINDS study had been conducted. "An even greater concern is that the effectiveness of thrombolysis in general community practice will be far less than any efficacy it achieved under the idealized circumstances of the NINDS trial."

Excellence would not, could not, in Hoffman's view, spread to ordinary emergency rooms. This brand of therapeutic pessimism, an article of faith that was to be controverted by numerous studies, developed into a serious obstacle. As more data emerged over the next decade, it would become clear that time-to-treatment was indeed highly significant, so that nothing but a CT scan ought to stand between a stroke patient and tPA. More patients did indeed benefit if they were treated within 90 minutes. But patients also did significantly better when treated between 90 minutes and 3 hours—indeed, it could eventually be shown, between 3 and as long as 4.5 hours. Making the drug effective in the community would mean—it means today—public education, universal fast recognition of stroke, and a whole evolving set of techniques for quick diagnosis.

In viewing the time window—the premise upon which the NINDS study was based—as the foremost stumbling block, Hoffman apparently depended solely on belief and epidemiological considerations. If he was familiar with the science underlying the decision to establish time-to-treatment, he did not in his publications cite or discuss it. The view that stroke was an acute emergency seemed not to be one Hoffman was willing to share. It was as if he did not want another clock in the busy emergency room—much less one located in the brain. But that meant in effect that he did not welcome a new era in stroke treatment; he hoped to close off an avenue he apparently believed was doomed to reach few patients while causing emergency physicians a surfeit of discomfort.

In addition to therapeutic pessimism, Hoffman's longstanding mistrust of drug companies also helped shape his views of tPA. He made revealing allusion, in the title of one of his op-ed pieces on tPA, to the famous fairy tale, "The Emperor's New Clothes." Hoffman's question, "And just what is the emperor of stroke wearing?" was a subtle, not to say clever, reminder of Genentech's original struggle to have tPA approved for heart attack.

It was a well-known story. In the 1980s, Genentech—grown rich and powered forward by a CEO from Big Pharma, Kirk Raabe—had been on the brink of gaining approval for tPA to treat heart attack when FDA scientists demanded evidence that the drug actually saved lives in clinical practice. About the same time, as described in Chapter 2, streptokinase returned to the clinic with a newly effective mode of administration. It was a double challenge. Hopeful that tPA might score a knockout against the older drug, Genentech funded a huge and expensive international trial—called GUSTO—that pitted the two treatments head-to-head. Although tPA emerged as significantly better than streptokinase, the difference between the two for heart attack was not as great as Genentech hoped or hyped. Now the emperor of clot-busters was said to be good for stroke and, wrote Hoffman, "[W]e should all ask why there's such a big parade and so many admirers of tPA's newest fancy clothes."

Hoffman's view of tPA as a pretender, undoubtedly due to this wider historical background, was another key to understanding his polemical stance. He was predisposed to distrust a clot-busting drug marketed by a powerful pharmaceutical company. Indeed, Hoffman claimed not to see why streptokinase, a far less expensive alternative, would not prove as effective. "[I]n the absence of studies directly comparing them, there is no reason to believe that tPA *should* be better than streptokinase for treating ischaemic stroke," wrote Hoffman in 2003. Yet he was fully aware that streptokinase had failed in each of three randomized stroke trials. Each had been terminated early due to excess deaths, including one that showed no benefit with a 3-hour time window.

Indeed, Hoffman might have known that available scientific evidence offered clear grounds for expecting that tPA would work better for stroke. Streptokinase provokes low blood pressure in about 1 in 10 patients, an undesirable event during an ischemic attack in the brain. In addition, it is less specific than tPA, which targets fibrin clots and thus reduces the potential for hemorrhage. Finally, streptokinase remains active in the bloodstream much longer than tPA. Conceivably, there might be an ideal dose and time-to-treatment window—but who was going to risk looking for it? Just that year, in 2000, Catherine Cornu and an international research team summed up the state of affairs: "Further trials with [streptokinase] could be justified, but the cost effectiveness and risks of pursuing such trials will need to be carefully weighed against the likelihood of improving on the benefits and costs of [tPA]." Nothing would change in the decade to come; no information would emerge to justify further trials with the older drug.

Hoffman did not always publish his articles in the most prominent journals— one of them appeared in a debate in the *Western Journal of Medicine* and another in an Australian medical journal—but his arguments received widespread attention from the emergency medicine community. Hoffman spoke out in his continuing medical education courses and put forth his views in debates and lectures. He took the controversy international. When other countries approved tPA for stroke, he often found a forum at which he could hope to influence emergency medicine communities outside the United States. He was an activist, working both within established professional societies and in unofficial venues such as his audiotapes series. He gathered supporters, some tenacious and vociferous, and he helped define the issue for the specialty as a whole.

Although the NINDS investigators, while the study was in progress, had little quarrel with Genentech, frustration with the company would eventually displace good feeling. For the trials, the company provided the drug and conducted itself credibly. Yet the researchers knew about Genentech's hyperactive marketing campaign on behalf of tPA for heart attack during the 1980s, so their concern for irreproachable ethical behavior ran high. Aware of the company's attention to stock prices and shareholders, when the trials were done, the leaders had quashed Genentech's hopes for early publicity prior to publication of the results in the *New England Journal of Medicine*. (The announcement, when it finally came, had no impact on stock prices.) But after the FDA approved the drug for stroke, the company conducted only the most anemic efforts to promote it. After advertising briefly in neurology journals, Genentech showed little interest and limited its efforts to educational programs. As drug companies often do, it had moved on to boost other leaders. The NINDS study investigators, after demanding restraint, ended up being disappointed with scant attention.

So it was a surprise in March 2002 when the *British Medical Journal* published a muckraking effort that attacked tPA for stroke: "Alteplase for Stroke: Money and Optimistic Claims Buttress the 'Brain Attack' Campaign." Written by Jeanne Lenzer, the article's several targets included the American Heart Association (AHA) for its endorsement of tPA, the physicians who drafted the AHA guidelines supporting use of the drug, and Genentech for corrupting the moral fiber of all concerned. Although narrowly focused on tPA for stroke, the article suggested it represented a prime example of the corrosive influence of pharmaceutical companies and of their unholy alliances forged with physicians and nonprofit organizations.

Much of the substance of Lenzer's story, which ran under the journal's rubric of "Education and debate," was hyperbole and old news. She absurdly claimed to be examining a conflict about a "treatment recommendation that could cost more lives than the disease itself." (All of the clinical trials showed no increase in bad outcomes, including death, in tPA-treated patients.) Two years earlier, investigative journalists who specialized in business-based malfeasance, Russell Mokhiber and Robert Weissman, had gleefully reported the essentials. The nonprofit AHA had taken large donations from Genentech and other large pharmaceutical firms. Genentech also contributed $2 million toward building a new conference center for the association. Did the famed biotech company receive more than a plaque to thank it for its contributions, which amounted to more than $10 million? Mohkiber and Weissman had no evidence but thought it must have. After initially giving tPA for stroke a tentative stamp of approval in 1997, in 2000 new practice guidelines from AHA upgraded the drug to "definitely recommended." Mokhiber and Weissman saw in this promotion an unmistakable *quid pro quo*. Their principal acknowledged informant was— Jerome Hoffman.

Lenzer now reported that seven of nine members on the AHA panel that reviewed the practice guidelines had some connection or other to Genentech. For whatever reason, whether through choice or due to editorial constraint, Lenzer did not name any of the panel members save Hoffman, who was one of the two panelists unconnected in any way to Genentech, and the lone dissenter. Lenzer channeled his distress and anger. He had apparently explained why he disagreed with the new recommendations in a letter to the AHA, but the organization declined to publish or even acknowledge it. This negligence, said Lenzer, "deprived the scientific community of knowledge about the basis for Dr. Hoffman's dissent and it obscured an important signal that any dissent existed at all."

Some of Lenzer's claims combined suspicion of misbehavior with Hoffman's therapeutic pessimism. She claimed the real impact of the drug could only be marginal, "with only 0.4% of patients potentially benefitting from [tPA]," a number in line with Hoffman's view that the drug could help at most 1 in 125 stroke patients. In like fashion, Lenzer criticized the "bloated claims" of the "brain attack" campaign that the AHA supported. "The term," she wrote, "was encouraged so clinicians and patients would think of stroke as an emergency on a par with myocardial infarction, or 'heart attack.'" That was precisely the idea—and a good one—but Lenzer, like Hoffman, viewed with suspicion the concept of stroke as an emergency. The "brain attack" campaign, she alleged, "rested on the touted value of alteplase."

Lenzer did not merely charge Genentech and the AHA with having "suppressed dissent" and "chameleon ethics" but also implicated the NINDS study itself. She repeated several of Hoffman's claims, including his suggestion that "chance alone could explain the benefit…". She did not acknowledge that the study consisted of two trials but, citing Hoffman, wrote that "critics caution that selective emphasis of a single study is scientific folly." That could be a fair statement, but here Lenzer ignored or distorted all supportive data. She dismissed one multihospital study, known as STARS, because Genentech supported it. She failed to mention studies of tPA in rural and community hospitals that indicated the drug could be successfully used outside academic settings. She paid no attention to highly positive results from Canada. Instead, she cited the retrospective chart study from Cleveland (see page 75) as evidence that community hospitals could not competently use tPA. What that research really showed was that hospitals and doctors should not ignore the same guidelines she criticized as bought and paid for.

In retrospect, a mixture of politics and the unique British experience with thrombolytic drugs was probably responsible for the appearance of Lenzer's article in a prestigious journal. Physicians in no country had given a cooler reception to tPA than England. There streptokinase had been extensively studied and owned a reputation as an inexpensive drug for heart attack that was essentially just as good as tPA. British neurologists were essentially uninvolved in stroke care, and the country had only marginal experience with emergency medicine as a specialty; the general practitioner took care of urgent cases. Lenzer's article would help choke off use of tPA in stroke in Britain for another 3 to 5 years.

Hoffman's critiques of the NINDS study and Lenzer's attacks, whatever their impact on slowing the adoption of tPA for stroke, certainly succeeded in sowing further confusion and doubt in the minds of emergency physicians in the United States. Among the debates, editorials, and flurry of letters published in the wake of the *British Medical Journal* article was one signed by James Li and five colleagues in emergency medicine. Li had helped Lenzer prepare her article; now in a separate missive he bemoaned the alleged risks of tPA. Contacted years later, he continues to think that physicians who believe the drug works are "suffering from the Hawthorne effect"—that is, they are psychologically disposed to believe the treatment is effective. He believes that "the true benefit of tPA is quite small" and its adverse effects "can be horrific."

For some number of emergency physicians, opposition to tPA for stroke became an article of faith. Still more adopted an attitude of hesitancy and uncertainty that persisted and percolated through the specialty. For some, reluctance to use tPA was due solely, and more or less legitimately, to lack of support from neurologists. Yet even under ideal conditions, according to a survey conducted in 2005, as many as two in five emergency physicians said they would not use tPA under any circumstances, owing mainly to the perceived risk of hemorrhage. It is fair to say that resistance in some places became part of the emergency medicine culture.

After her article in the *British Medical Journal* "sparked off controversy," Lenzer took credit for provoking a full re-analysis of the NINDS data by a wholly independent panel of eminent biostatisticians. But the results of this undertaking, published in 2004, she did not like: they fully supported the original NINDS study. So Lenzer published a new article that repeatedly cited Hoffman, who rehashed his concerns about "baseline imbalances." She also apparently talked with emergency physician David Schriger, who cast his objections to the re-analysis in a uniquely rhetorical way.

"Imagine you are underneath two airplanes," explained Shriger, a colleague of Hoffman's at UCLA, "that cross directly above you at different altitudes. You might think they collided. So might someone standing a few feet away from you. Someone in a third plane at the same altitude as one of the others would be quite certain that no collision occurred." Schriger explained the relevance of all this with a rare example of anthropomorphizing in epidemiology. "The original NINDS analysis and the re-analysis are like the two people," he explained, "who are standing near each other. They confirm that from that perspective it appears that the drug may be efficacious, but not necessarily effective."

This tendentious argument actually holds an important lesson about statistical evaluations and science in medicine. Hoffman and Lenzer, Schriger, and others who became late critics of tPA for stroke, relied invariably and exclusively on clinical epidemiology, sometimes annealed to personal passion. The various studies of patients—randomized, observational, retrospective—were the sole sources of information they cited; they ignored the underlying science entirely. This left them in the end with nothing but guesswork, doubts, and hints of dark external forces shaping the numbers. Epidemiology provides powerful tools for confirming or falsifying hypotheses about whether a treatment is effective, but it is only through the deductive tools of science—biochemistry, animal studies, physiology—that these hypotheses arise at all. To ignore the science that brings about clinical trials is fatal to what is popularly called "evidence-based medicine"—that is, the use of basic science and clinical trials to evaluate treatments.

In retrospect, the 2004 re-analysis of the NINDS study probably marks the date after which skepticism as to whether tPA worked was no longer tenable. That year also saw publication of a "pooled analysis." This analysis of the NINDS study together with the other randomized trials, five in all, showed once more that the treatment was effective and also indicated that the window might be extended to 4.5 hours from symptom onset. This finding became the basis of another incarnation of the European Cooperative Acute Stroke Study (ECASS III).

As major new studies returned now-predictable results about the effectiveness of tPA in treating strokes of all kinds, Jerome Hoffman discovered what he perceived as crucial flaws in every one of them. After the 2004 pooled analysis, Hoffman again brought up streptokinase and the heart attack trials and called for the NINDS trial to be replicated. In 2009, after completion of ECASS III, Hoffman viewed it "as not designed, however, to confirm or disconfirm the results of the only prior 'positive' [NINDS] study, and its results are markedly different than those of every other previous RCT conducted in patients treated more than 3 hours after symptom onset." But useful comparisons could indeed be made, and assertions to the contrary wore thin.

For her part, Jeanne Lenzer continued periodically to revisit tPA for stroke, always with a jaundiced eye for the drug and a tender word for her intellectual accomplice. In 2005 she published an article entitled "The New Alchemy" that discussed tPA for stroke as a cautionary tale for journalists who ought, she wrote, to "stop acting as lapdogs for the scientific community and start acting as watchdogs." Three years later, in a popular magazine, she published a story about a doctor who administered tPA to a patient who died from a hemorrhage, so she claimed, "not from his stroke but from effects of tPA, the drug that was meant to save him." Phillip A. Brewer, the doctor in question, was upset and confused. "So, like many physicians, he turned to the articles and analyses of Jerome Hoffman," an "elder statesman of medicine." Explained Brewer: "Dr. Hoffman has a brilliant mind. He is listened to and trusted by more emergency physicians than anyone I know."

But this was rearguard action, small beer, pure hagiography, and no longer the *British Medical Journal* but *Discover* magazine. It was unfortunate and in some ways it was sad: neither Hoffman nor Lenzer wanted to acknowledge at long last that tPA had been a poor example of the "hidden hand of industry." They wanted still to see in it rapacious Big Pharma manipulating physicians and nonprofits and the kind of "checkbook science" that purchased recommendations, guidelines, and prescriptions.

Oddly enough, Hoffman himself had described better than anyone the fate awaiting his views on tPA and stroke. In 2000, in collaboration with Katherine Callen King, a professor of classics and comparative literature, he had inaugurated what he hoped would become an ongoing series called "Myths and Medicine" in the *Western Journal of Medicine*. "When myths convince us to act in ways that are contrary to our own interests, or (for healers) to the interests of patients," the authors wrote, "we must first recognize them for what they are, then critically challenge their assumptions, and finally, have the courage to abandon them."

By 2010 many were waiting, few were expecting. But in fact the game was up, for countervailing forces were catching up with negative spin about tPA. Approval in Canada in 1999 led to fairly extensive use, absent universal public awareness. In the United Kingdom and the European Union, by contrast, approval only in 2002 set the stage for infrastructure reforms in a number of countries. The considerable and expanding literature on tPA for stroke included novel and intriguing avenues. They showed the drug worked in many venues and different kinds of patients. Numerous studies confirmed that rural hospitals could successfully use tPA without heightened risk of hemorrhage or mortality. There were case reports of tPA successfully administered to a 15-year-old girl and a 103-year-old woman.

Inside emergency medicine, from about 2003 onward, there was gradual realignment, a softening of resistance that moved toward a tipping point by the end of the first decade of the new millennium. If in 2009 you were an emergency doctor, you probably belonged to its guild-like organization, the American College of Emergency Physicians. You would have heard that the guidelines concerning tPA for stroke were being redrafted—and in conjunction, no less, with the American Academy of Neurology. If you worked at a university medical center and also belonged to the Society of Academic Emergency Physicians (SAEM), you would have learned that, also in 2009, the organization rescinded its statement on tPA, which had been in place for some 8 years. In a letter made public, the organization's Board of Directors seemed pleased, perhaps relieved, to sundown the old, negative-tinged policy. Results from the ECASS III, which suggested a 4.5-hour window might be workable, seemed to be the final straw.

"The time is ripe for a change," said Yu-Feng Yvonne Chan, an assistant professor of emergency medicine who led the organization's Neurological Interest Group. "Those of us in SAEM pride ourselves on being on the cutting edge of research, and on being more evidence-based."

A movement in favor of tPA for stroke was visible both on collective and individual levels, with a growing understanding of stroke as an acute emergency. Other organizations have emerged to advance emergency medicine in caring for urgent neurological conditions, both in terms of original research and training of physicians. The Neurological Emergencies Treatment Trials (NETT) Network was established by Bill Barsan, with considerable funding from NINDS; the Foundation for Education and Research in Neurological Emergencies (FERNE) was founded in 1997 in the wake of the NINDS trials, and it has actively campaigned for acceptance of tPA for stroke.

Younger doctors also reflect a growing climate of acceptance. "If you go to a resident-based meeting," says Andy Jagoda, a FERNE founder and chairman of the Department of Emergency Medicine at Mt. Sinai Hospital in New York, "almost all the residents will raise their hands: they believe in tPA for stroke."

But resistance abided. It came to center around the idea that clot-busting therapy should be considered "standard of care"—a term with both institutional and legal ramifications. Emergency physician and professor Robert M. McNamara, in his 2009 article in the *Annals of Emergency Medicine*, repeated many of Jerome Hoffman's criticisms of tPA for stroke, adding an element of self-flagellation. "We know that despite our efforts," he wrote, citing a 15-year-old study, "often we are simply not good at diagnosing stroke." He hoped emergency doctors would resist the "you can do it" attitude pressed upon them, and he wrote: "I believe we need to declare a moratorium on the efforts to make this therapy the expected 'standard of care' in community hospitals."

This was an appeal without substance, according to Andy Jagoda. He qualified McNamara's objections as "just empty talk." He was frankly dismissive. "Because [tPA] *is* standard of care. You can't get around it. You just can't. It's FDA-approved. We have a whole stroke center initiative in America. We have 25% of hospitals endorsing its use. We have the major certifying body, the Joint Commission, endorsing its use. It's being looked at as a core measure by [the Centers for Medicare and Medicaid Services]. It's just stupid. You might not agree with it. You might read the literature differently. But to say that it's not standard of care is just putting your head in the sand."

In science and medicine, anachronistic beliefs are nothing new. It took a long time—about 15 years, in fact—for physicians to come to a consensus about the dangers of smoking. Belief in eugenics, confidence in the health benefits of megadose vitamins, and conviction that schizophrenia was caused by bad mothering are all testament to the power of temperament and stubborn convictions that enable scientists of every caliber to hold views long past the time that they are plausible or even taken seriously. With tPA for stroke there comes into contention not just a theory but a set of facts about the only effective treatment for a common and dangerous disease that grievously afflicts the brain and every year irreparably harms millions of people.

Money and Brains | 7

*T*he 21st century should have brought good news for victims of ischemic stroke. The original National Institute of Neurological Disorders and Stroke (NINDS) study had several times been reaffirmed, and the safety and efficacy of tPA ensured. Controversy, some perhaps inevitable and more of it unnecessary, had retarded acceptance of the drug while a virulent debate roiled neurology. The situation eventually clarified to the extent that, as the editorial in the journal *Stroke* declared, "Enough is enough!" By then, about 2002, only a hard core of skeptical neurologists remained unconvinced of tPA's effectiveness, even if some stayed permanently sour as to whether large numbers of patients could recognize stroke symptoms and seek treatment fast.

Yet tPA remained vastly underused. Just about 2% of acute stroke patients received it, although in principle as many as 50% might benefit. The best overall explanation for this disparity is, in a word, money.

With tPA for stroke, money has its own Rashomon-like story to tell and lives up to its characterization as the great motivator. The NINDS study researchers began to see that in a real sense the failure to implement tPA, especially as it persisted, was largely about money. They cited paltry payments from Medicare for hospitals and nonexistent supplemental compensation for doctors, all in addition to chronic lack of funds to promote public awareness.

Inadequate reimbursement became a serious disincentive to use tPA on stroke patients and, perversely, the cost in damaged brains has been incalculable.

The money issue was significant in a particular way. Stroke qualifies as "low profile" compared with many diseases that are *not* so much about money. Research funds for some disorders are abundant even while results have been virtually negligible over the course of decades and generations. Many lethal cancers fall into this category, as do various severe genetic disorders. Money enough cannot keep oncologists, today as yesterday, from having to admit their inability to effectively treat tumors of brain and spine, lungs, pancreas, and liver. Similarly, research into genetic disorders such as cystic fibrosis has been heavily funded by activist communities of victims and their families, but to little avail. Not mammon but a dearth of knowledge around complex cellular dynamics is responsible for the meager therapeutic yield.

For stroke, by contrast, once tPA had been shown to work, the challenge was to generate and diffuse knowledge about it in both public and professional spheres, to effect substantial changes in perception, and to improve the medical community's aptitude for action. That would require abundant funding from which stroke had never benefitted.

Zivin started hearing about the problem, as it affected doctors and hospitals, only in fits and starts. For a long time, he and most of the NINDS study researchers remained ignorant of its magnitude. This owed, in retrospect, to fog surrounding the Ivory Tower: they were all academics and not exposed to the types of financial pressures as people in private practice. They were blindsided by the kinds of problems tPA faced as it moved into the marketplace.

At Veterans Hospital in San Diego, private-practice neurologists would sometimes come to the clinics Zivin ran, and in talking with them he started to recognize the scope of the problem. He would ask them, "How are things? What's going on in your hospital?" They would start to complain. They were not receiving decent or extra compensation for acute stroke. They were not prepared for the emergency call. The hospital was not giving them any reimbursement for that.

On reflection, the fact that the NINDS study researchers were forced to scale back expectations in the short term was not surprising. They had to adjust to the idea that their hopes for tPA would not be soon met in any respect, that it would take time measured in years for the medicine to be adopted, for awareness to be raised, and for use to increase. From their highly invested and personal standpoint, it was hard to understand why. Several years would pass before reality sank in.

The trouble started with Genentech. The biotech firm's failure to spend heavily to market tPA for stroke was a blow the significance of which can only be guessed. After approval, the company took out a modest series of advertisements in the neurology journals. This campaign lasted about 6 months and died without discernible impact.

The slick pages of Genentech's annual report for 1996, the year that tPA was approved for stroke, were revealing. The company relegated the clot-buster to second place, behind its growth hormone products. Colorful thick-coated pages with photo montages displayed the drugs as equals, although one of them was for dwarfism, a rare condition, while the other treated the third most common cause of death and the leading cause of severe disability.

Indeed, their only genuine commonality was that both drugs chased profits for Genentech. Nutropin was "for the long-term treatment of short stature," a chromosomal disorder that could now be addressed by administering daily injections for years. Furthermore, Nutropin was used every day, whereas tPA was used once. Even a modestly priced daily treatment eventually generates more income than a high-priced single treatment.

But the issue of money ran deeper and was more pervasive than Genentech's search for profits. Nutropin was one result of the Orphan Drug Act, enacted in 1983 to offer pharmaceutical firms extended patent protection and tax incentives to create drugs for rare diseases. Once approved, moreover, growth hormone could be prescribed to treat not only "short stature" but the narrower category of dwarfism. With its medicine for these disorders Genentech in 1996 claimed a two-thirds market share. A photo showed 18-year-old Maisha Lauer, whose predicted height was well below normal. Instead she was almost 5 feet tall, presumably thanks to Nutropin.

The headline for stroke, by contrast, pointed out, "The Message is Urgency." A squib discussed company salesmen working toward a treatment protocol at St. Anthony's Hospital in the small farm town of Effingham, Illinois. A photo showed 67-year-old Rosetta Bolander, who had suffered a stroke but "recovered with no signs of damage, much to the delight of her six children, 17 grandchildren and two great grandchildren." She had sought treatment fast because she had seen reports of tPA on television. There was no discussion of prospective market or market share.

"I think the company made a very big mistake at the beginning," recalled Tom Brott, the NINDS investigator who had run the successful rapid response program in Cincinnati. At the time, he suggested that Genentech help support a 300-patient study to investigate whether tPA worked at a lower dose, perhaps with less risk of hemorrhage. Such a study would be ethical, raise awareness of the drug, and clear up concern over safety. "It was," said Brott, "a win-win for the company." But the company was not buying: it had not paid for the NIH-sponsored NINDS study and was not going to start funding clinical trials now.

"They initially helped us put together some educational materials for emergency physicians," remembered Jim Grotta. "But they basically looked at what they had anticipated sales were going to be, and said, 'We're never going to make enough money from this drug.'"

Although not predictable, the Genentech decision to not aggressively develop a market for stroke predated the NINDS studies. Elliott Grossbard, after all, had initially rejected Zivin's earliest request for tPA in 1983 and cited his training with preeminent neurologist Raymond Adams of Massachusetts General Hospital, who "told us that stroke is not treatable." This negative attitude persisted within Genentech on the business side even as stroke became a target for tPA, and it was evidently still preponderant more than a decade later. For all that Genentech saw itself at the cutting edge of biotech, full of promise for the future of medicine, it seemed as if the marketplace outweighed its aspirations to treat one of the most serious diseases of mankind. The company would do nothing of substance to change anachronistic attitudes toward stroke, whether among doctors or patients.

The level of support that Genentech provided tPA for stroke was in stark contrast to the company's pioneering enthusiasm concerning the drug's use for heart attack. In the late 1980s, while under development, tPA represented the firm's great promise. It was, according to Genentech CEO Kirk Raab, "the driving force to give the company its heroic dimensions." Hoping to make tPA a revolutionary treatment for heart attack, it spent lavishly to market the drug both before and after FDA approval. When ambiguity over efficacy loomed, the company helped fund the Global Utilization of Streptokinase and Tissue Plasminogen Activator to Treat Occluded Arteries, known as GUSTO, the huge trial that narrowly but decisively proved tPA saved more lives than its less costly rival, streptokinase.

The NINDS study investigators could be forgiven their disappointment with Genentech if they recalled that, just a month after FDA approval of tPA for heart attack in 1988, hospitals were falling over one another to obtain the drug. One pharmacist at the time called it a "stampede" with such strong sales due to Genentech's "tremendous job of pre-marketing…so that the cardiologists are salivating." Indeed, Genentech was accused of over-zealous salesmanship and brazen tactics, of warning about a possible tPA shortage in order to spur sales. Raab would always defend the huge promotional outlay. It "showed to the physician community, the cardiologists, that we were behind the product. We spent sixty million dollars to do a trial [GUSTO] that big, and that's putting your money where you mouth is."

Nothing like that happened with stroke.

It should be noted that by 1996 Genentech had nearly 15 years of experience with the drug, not all of it positive. Even as a moneymaker for myocardial infarction, it had not performed as well as hoped. Genentech waged patent wars, tPA battled other treatments, and company stock suffered. It was painful, recalled Herbert Heyneker, one of the main molecular biologists at Genentech, "to see it stall around a hundred and fifty million," lower than predicted by a factor of seven. "I think that market acceptance and market introduction were slower than projected." It did not help that the high price created resentment among some doctors even as the cost ($2,200) was stoutly defended by executives and, truth to tell, today might be considered a bargain—particularly in light of comparable surgical therapies such as angioplasty and stenting.

Another reason Genentech gave short shrift to tPA for stroke reflected the uncomfortable alliance between academic "thought leaders" and biotech companies seeking to maximize revenues. For all that the NINDS study researchers all now advocated tPA after conclusion of the randomized trials, as individuals and a group they kept their distance from Genentech. The regulatory climate demanded it to some extent. So they had responded negatively, for instance, when company executives floated the idea of announcing the results prior to publication of the famous paper in the *New England Journal of Medicine*.

"We told them we'd take them to the mat," said Tom Brott. By this maneuver, he believed, Genentech only hoped to burnish its stock price. In fact, with the drug already on the market for heart disease and now approved for stroke, immediate promulgation of the message would not have been at all out of place or unethical. In retrospect at least, the NINDS study researchers' rectitude may be understood as misplaced. As it turned out, it was another ingredient in a recipe for neglect.

Finally, and perhaps most importantly, there was no advocate (or champion) for tPA within Genentech itself in 1996. Executives were negative and skeptical. "They didn't think there was going to be a market to sell very much tPA because of the time window," said Bill Bennett, a senior scientist who at the time was working on a second-generation version of the drug. Spending large sums to heighten public awareness of stroke seemed like an extra step with an uncertain return. It had been unnecessary with tPA for heart attack, the disease around which much of emergency medicine had been developed over the course of a generation.

"We didn't have what you would call an internal cheerleader for stroke who could muster the enthusiasm we had for myocardial infarction," said Bennett. This final contingent fact was significant. In the end, none of the Genentech executives shared the enthusiasm of the NINDS study researchers, never had, and so the considerable attention that might be gained through extensive and targeted advertising would not be forthcoming.

It is fair to speculate that Genentech's decision to not aggressively market tPA seriously affected how doctors and healthcare providers perceived the drug and how often it was used. But the victims of this neglect were the people who suffered ischemic stroke. For them, awareness of symptoms and signs was of prime importance. Even more than heart attack, clots and clogged arteries in the brain do not telegraph their presence by aches, pains, or fevers. Stroke is so sudden, and prompt treatment so important for a good outcome, that preloaded sensitivity is crucial. There, too, effective and sustained advertising from Genentech could have helped.

In terms of money, the broader background was equally important. Pharmaceutical advertising budgets changed radically in the late 1990s, just about the time tPA for stroke won approval. In 1997, just a year later, the FDA fostered a rapid upsurge in drug advertising on television, leading to the direct-to-consumer (DTC) model that has since become integral to the healthcare marketing landscape, for better or worse. Today pharmaceutical firms are regularly attacked for overselling their products to a mass audience.

But tPA for stroke has never enjoyed such attention—with some irony. Unlike sleeping tablets or cholesterol-lowering medication, it is not taken on daily basis. It is the furthest thing from a lifestyle drug like Viagra for impotence or Rogaine for baldness. Although knowledge about it should reach the largest possible audience, it does not fit the consumer model for drugs that sell to the masses.

In addition to marketing was the issue of compensation for hospitals and doctors. Medicare reimbursement rates did not change with the advent of tPA but remained etched in stone, and over time these became powerful impediments to the drug's wider use. They helped ensure its marginalization even after numerous research papers confirmed its safety. In addition, underuse led to a lack of appreciation of tPA's cost-saving benefits.

Patients with acute stroke who do not receive tPA do not generally pose a heavy financial burden for hospitals. When patients arrive in the emergency room, evaluation may be extensive, with imaging studies and blood chemistry and neurological workups. But treatment—if tPA is off the table—is most often only supportive: blood pressure monitored, intravenous fluids to avoid dehydration. Such patients can be bedded in corridors and ignored for hours or even days (see Chapter 8). Hospitals do not go broke by providing this level of treatment. Nor will they lose money by giving tPA to the exceptional patient with clear-cut symptoms who happens to arrive in the emergency department with instant dispatch and finds an able staff and willing physician.

By contrast, a dedicated acute stroke team that aims at proactive use of tPA costs substantially more. Emergency personnel trained to treat stroke must be on hand at all times, able to rapidly evaluate patients as they arrive, with no time to spare. Someone, usually a nurse, must be ready to transport the patient to the imaging suite, where a technician is needed to operate the CT scanner. A radiologist must be available to read the images while, ideally, a neurologist assesses the patient and makes the differential diagnosis. For administration, tPA must be mixed to order and liquefied from solid form, which means a pharmacist may be involved, although today this task often belongs to a nurse. Empirically, too, as treatment has evolved, hospital stays for stroke patients who do receive tPA can be longer because these patients tend to be sicker. To the cost of all the above, add approximately $2,000, the bare price for the drug.

One may ask: is such care not reimbursed by insurance? Expensive treatments abound in today's medicine; are not most of them covered by third-party payers? Surely, stroke is covered. Why should we argue that stroke is under-reimbursed when nobody complains much about payment for all manner of, say, emergency intervention for heart attack?

In fact, hospitals are sensitive to costs and inadequate reimbursement for specific diseases, diagnostic tests, and procedures—to everything that affects care and reaches the bottom line. Low compensation for stroke owes in the first instance to the historical inability to treat, and it represents a blockading inertial force. Patients shuttled into a corner of the emergency room, with physical signs stabilized while their brains lose about 2 million neurons each minute (not to mention 14 billion synapses) do not cost much. While trained caregivers treat heart attack with a host of interventions, nothing significantly bettered the treatment of acute stroke until the advent of tPA.

The most authoritative arbiter for reimbursement is the Centers for Medicare and Medicaid Services (CMS), the *de facto* adjudicator for insurance payouts under federal programs. Since it was established in the 1960s, CMS has employed diagnosis-related groups, or DRGs, to decide on dollar amounts that hospitals receive for services provided. This influential system, also widely adopted in Europe as a cost-containment strategy, provides fixed sums for specific diagnoses, regardless of how much care any individual patient requires or receives. Part of the rationale for such a system is that costs for a given disorder will average out across large numbers of patients. Without entering into details—an entire profession of coding specialists has grown up around DRGs—hospitals thus bill Medicare for each eligible emergency, including, for stroke, "intracranial hemorrhage or cerebral infarction."

Until recently, the associated reimbursement was under $6,000. The advent of tPA, in 1997, did not provoke CMS to change its payout, which remained roughly the same over the next 10 years. To give patients the only drug available to clear brains of clogged blood vessels thus became medically sound but, in the short term, financially unwise.

Similarly, CMS also determined compensation for attending physicians, and there the situation was and continues to be still worse. Reimbursement for doctors treating stroke in 2002, for example, whether they provided the drug or not, was about $450. Spend an hour, spend a day or night with the patient, and the doctor receives globally the same amount. A code was eventually created for thrombolysis (clot-busting), but the added reimbursement was— zero. Doctors administering tPA, with its value-added calculus of risks versus benefits, received the same money as if they had given the patient aspirin or a sugar pill.

For doctors and hospitals alike, these were strong disincentives. Neurologists in private practice are small businessmen, and hospitals are usually corporations. Although doctors are dedicated to helping the sick, and hospitals often have diverse sources of revenue, neither can afford to lose money on a consistent basis for a particular disease.

To be sure, some hospitals and neurologists understood and tried to address these issues. Most of the NINDS study researchers themselves were neurologists who helped constitute beachhead communities that understood tPA. Often they had worked for these hospitals and had participated in the NINDS trials and were committed to treating complex cases. "You had some hospitals that were doing the right thing," said Joe Broderick, "spending the resources, but actually losing money on every [stroke] patient who came in." At other institutions, tPA for stroke was neither here nor there, "not on the radar screen" of hospital administrators. At these places stroke continued to be treated as it always had been—with tender, loving nothing.

In what was turning into the looking-glass logic of acute stroke therapy, tPA was not only dramatically underused and severely undercompensated, it also saved money. Research on the costs and benefits of tPA for stroke started almost as soon as it came to market, and was later replicated. This brings the story up to the present—leading to a final and increasingly urgent reason, as we will see, why physicians and hospitals should treat acute stroke with tPA and why the public at large should be aware of it.

In 1998, little more than a year after FDA approval, Susan C. Fagan and a number of NINDS colleagues published an article in *Neurology* that examined the economics surrounding tPA. Did tPA for stroke, an expensive treatment in and of itself, save money? Extrapolating data from the NINDS study, they estimated costs for 1,000 patients treated with tPA compared with the same number declared ineligible for the drug. The average length of hospital stay turned out to be a day and a half shorter for the tPA group, and a higher percentage of these patients—fully one-third more—returned home instead of being shuttled to long-term care facilities. The higher costs of acute care (in aggregate about $2 million for every 1,000 patients treated) were more than offset by reduced costs for rehabilitation ($2 million) and nursing homes ($4.8 million). The greater cost for tPA patients during the first hospitalization was recouped within a year.

In their essentials, these results have been confirmed time and again. They have never been controverted. Recent studies include the concept of quality-adjusted life years (QALYs), a means of computing the value of a specific treatment based on the caliber of life it confers on survivors over time. Weighting the quality of post-stroke life, Susan Fagan points to a recent study by Danish economist Lars Ehrlers and colleagues that shows that the entire cost of setting up a stroke center to provide tPA, including the cost of a CT scanner, is recoverable within a year. This model, she points out, "saved money and saved QALYs."

As the exceptional "cost-effective" drug, tPA improves quality of life *and* reduces overall medical costs. Most medical interventions aim at improving lives, whether short term or long term. The various drugs known as proton pump inhibitors, for example, may relieve last night's acid reflux, while a hip replacement keeps people walking for years. Both are worthwhile, yet neither reduces the overall cost of illness. But tPA, in relieving acute congestion in the brain with sustainable results, both avoids permanent damage and mitigates cost.

Many of the NINDS study researchers worked on the cost-analysis issue, and their publications were eventually augmented by others, both in the United States and internationally. Analyses conducted in the United Kingdom, Canada, and Denmark all showed cost savings and cost effectiveness compared with doing nothing. By 2007 Terence J. Quinn and colleagues in Glasgow, Scotland, could write, counter to much opinion in England, that the "results of economic analysis are unanimously in favor of tPA use when the wider implications of reduced disability are considered."

For hospitals, Medicare reimbursement eventually did increase, and this positive outcome owed in part to all the studies demonstrating cost-effectiveness. In late 2005, pressure on CMS officials from the American Stroke Association, the Brain Attack Coalition, and other groups, together with data from Medicare's own database, known as MedPAR, finally bore fruit. CMS created a category for thrombolysis (clot-busting) that effectively doubled the average payout, from a little under $6,000 to $11,578.

This significant adjustment came with severe limitations, however. Physicians are still under-compensated; nothing has changed there. And more money for hospitals, though it might raise awareness of tPA among administrators and win the attention of emergency room personnel, could of itself do little to undo the damage a decade of neglect had wrought. It was an advance but not more than a first step toward reconciling a powerful treatment with the financial incentive for using it.

Even if it did not save money, tPA would still be worth using. Cost-effectiveness is a helpful tool for parsing the rationale underlying medical interventions. But as a concept it had been invented and was useful in correcting "distortions" in a regulated marketplace such as health care, not as an end in itself. Drilling down deeper, what cost analysis really points to is how clearly and consistently thrombolytic therapy saves brains. In terms of net risk, dissolving clots within a specific timeframe does not make strokes worse or lead to greater (and costly) disability.

When Zivin and colleagues were developing it, they worried about this possibility. They knew what stroke could do, but what about tPA? Could it make a survivable ischemic stroke worse? Many patients recover with only "minor" paralysis, for example, with bearable limitations to movement and cognitive impairment. Mild deficits might entail only anger, frustration, and depression—if that. But catastrophic stroke can leave victims immobilized, lacking the sensation of touch, unable to recognize their own limbs. They may suffer pain untreatable even with today's drugs. Worse still, aphasia can deprive patients of the ability to use language or comprehend it. Many stroke victims become unable to wash themselves, put on their clothes, or control bowel and bladder. They suffer personality change and dementia. They may lapse into a vegetative state with no chance of recovery. Saving lives only to create such conditions is not desirable. An additional positive outcome of the NINDS study was to show that tPA precisely did not create these kinds of cases. The drug instead saved patients from what most people would agree is a fate worse than death.

This fact has recently started to create a new understanding and appreciation of the post-stroke victim, of the paralyzed and debilitated patient. Failure to administer tPA in appropriate circumstances is changing the way some patients and families view the outcome. In today's conflicted health care climate, this shift is bound to affect both doctors and hospitals. As exaggerated anxieties about the risk of cerebral hemorrhage recede, essentially invalidating the fears of emergency physicians, tPA is charting a course toward acceptance, especially at major medical centers, as the "standard of care" for patients who meet the simple requirements of protocol.

But today the drug is becoming "all about money" in yet another way. Patients who feel deprived, and their families, have resorted to legal measures: they have sued. Resistance to tPA, long buffeted by financial disincentives to treat, has at last spawned what nobody wanted—charges of liability, malpractice, and lawsuits over stroke damage—in short, a legal dilemma.

Deer in the Headlights | 8

*U*pset himself and anxious, Don Mead did not understand at first. His wife Judy was agitated in addition to everything else. As they sped to the hospital, she balefully eyed the steering wheel, lifted her left arm, and made guttural sounds. It was "one of the those crazy things you'll remember forever." Not 10 minutes before, Judy had been a healthy 49-year-old woman. Now she was having a stroke.

An ordinary morning in August 2009, gone suddenly haywire. At their ranch in Santa Barbara County, California, Don and Judy raised wild boar, boarded horses, and supplied exotic meats to local restaurants. Routine dominates life with livestock, so every midweek morning Don rose early and brewed coffee while Judy slept an extra few minutes. Invariably he waited for her at the foot of the stairs when she came down, to lift her past the first step. It was a romantic gesture after 10 years of marriage. Judy was small beside Don, her size offset by a big smile and oval face; she had brown eyes and auburn hair. That morning, as usual, they breakfasted in the living room, sitting close together on the couch, touching as they always did, and talking for about 20 minutes. Then Don took a quick shower and dressed. Nothing was amiss until, as he came downstairs, strange noises came from the kitchen. There he found her.

Judy lay sprawled on the floor, in her housecoat, face down.

She had been putting away the dishes. A plate was misplaced, wedged halfway out of a stack in the cupboard. Judy must have fallen that suddenly. When Don turned her over, her gaze told him what was happening.

"It was apparent right away that it was a stroke," Don recalls. He hoped she might have merely fainted but what little he knew left no doubt. "A lot of people say the face sags but it does not; it just doesn't operate the way it used to; it doesn't work right."

In addition to the facial droop, Judy had lost the ability to speak. "She was trying to talk but all that would come out were these guttural sounds."

What Don happened to know about stroke was simple, elementary, and correct. He had gleaned the essentials from nothing more than reading magazines. The concept of a "clot-buster" drug was easy to grasp and it stuck with him. His life in farming and animal husbandry undoubtedly helped.

"What always struck me is the name is very catchy because of the *Ghostbusters* movie."

Too, he knew clot-busters had to happen fast. Fortunately, or so it seemed. The nearest hospital, Lompoc Valley Medical Center, was just a 10-minute drive from the ranch. Don carried Judy to the truck. He drove above the speed limit, phoning the California Highway Patrol to alert them. He also requested they inform the emergency service at the hospital: he was bringing in a stroke victim.

Only after a moment did Don recognize the object of Judy's acute distress, the meaning of the sounds she was making and her gesture, lifting her arm. The emergency blinkers. Their repetitive tick-tock sound vexed and annoyed her. He shut them off. Judy's relief was sudden and evident.

Arriving at the hospital within minutes of an ischemic stroke makes most patients excellent candidates for tPA; and the sooner they receive it, the greater their chances for the best possible recovery. It ought to have helped, too, that Don made it clear, from the first moment he spoke with the doctor: he wanted Judy to get the "clot-busters" he had read about. But he was willing to be instructed.

"The doctor told me clot-busters couldn't be used until they were sure she wasn't bleeding internally," said Don. "And that was why they were going to rush her off to a CT scan."

Lompoc Valley Medical Center had a stroke protocol that included use of tPA. By the time the radiologist called to say there was no bleed, Judy had undergone basic triage by the nurses and assessment by Dr. Sadaf Khan, the emergency room physician. Dr. Khan's neurological exam noted Judy's unresponsiveness on the right side of her body and her right facial droop. Although she noted Judy did not speak, in her notes she did not specifically use the medical term, aphasia.

The symptoms pointed to stroke even though Judy was relatively young. For reasons that would never become clear, that diagnosis was not made at this point. The doctor had started to act according to the rules for administering tPA but did not follow through. She later said she had given the drug several times at other institutions but did not recall having read the Lompoc Valley Community Hospital protocol for its use. She might in any event have gone ahead to give the drug once the CT results were available. But she did not. Instead, she ran more tests. An hour passed. A lumbar puncture of the spine confirmed: no bleeding in Judy's brain stem; that would have signaled another type of event, called a subarachnoid hemorrhage. But now what?

As minutes passed, Don grew by turns restless, annoyed, and angry. Most of all, he got scared. He had been with his wife every moment since finding her in the kitchen. At the hospital entrance he was grateful for the wheelchair the nurses brought to take Judy into the emergency room. They disrobed her and placed her on a bed. She resisted, upset and angry. She was unable to speak but Don could read the distress and confusion in her gaze. Now the second hour ticked away.

"The whole thing was going along at a crazy rate for me because I was getting pretty distressed at that point."

Although the CT scan did not indicate a bleeding stroke and Judy was still within the three-hour window to receive tPA, Dr. Khan sought help, late in the morning, from a neurologist. She believed she had detected spontaneous movement in Judy's right lower extremity and perhaps her right upper extremity. Although this kind of "improvement" would not in and of itself contraindicate treatment with tPA, she now called Dr. Phillip Ente. On staff at the hospital, Ente was that morning in his satellite office about twenty miles away from Lompoc. He spoke to Dr. Khan on the telephone but did not come to the emergency room. He asked her to perform certain tests to measure what she suggested was improvement in Judy's condition and then he helped Dr. Khan decide. She soon wrote it down, as she acknowledged: "no Lytics, already improving neurologically."

Judy would not receive tPA.

"I had given my faith over to the doctor to do what she needed to do," recalled Don ruefully. "When I asked for clot-busters I didn't know she had to be checked for bleeding. Because that wasn't a layman thing. I thought: They have to do what they have to do."

The time window for giving the drug passed.

Whether Don was informed of the decision not to use tPA would also be in dispute. He was, he says, told nothing. He claimed he had specifically requested clot-busters and continued to ask about them into the afternoon, long after the possibility of giving tPA was gone. Dr. Khan's only notes concerning the consultation with the neurologist read: "Discussed with Dr. Ente regarding MRI. He will see tomorrow." And she added her comment about "No lytics." She made no notation of having informed Don of her decision.

Judy had been provided the classic treatment for stroke. That is, she received nothing.

Meanwhile, as noontime passed, Don was instructed to return to his ranch, to search the medicine chest and report back on any medications Judy might be using. While still hoping Judy might receive tPA, Don complied but later called this mission nothing but "chores" because he knew she wasn't taking anything except the usual bunch of vitamins. He dutifully carried them back to the hospital pharmacy as asked—but it made no difference.

In the afternoon of the day of her stroke, care for Judy was transferred to Celia Ramos, who would become her primary care physician. By 2 o'clock in the afternoon Judy had been wheeled off to one of the hospital's regular rooms and hooked up to an IV for nourishment. She was provided no medication that might improve her condition. Nothing, by then, would have done any good.

Judy Mead continued to receive nothing—at least, nothing specific for stroke—for the next 6 days. She did not recover the ability to speak and remained paralyzed on one side of her body. Don stayed with her. He slept next to her bed in the bare room of the single-story hospital. He telephoned Gina, Judy's daughter from her first marriage, who flew out to California and stayed at the ranch. The first time she came to the hospital, Judy broke into a huge smile—with half her mouth.

Others came to Judy's bedside. Her best friend, Annise Spangler, sat with her regularly and spelled Don so he could return to the ranch to take care of a minimum of business. She helped feed Judy, and talked to her, tried to read to her, lift her spirits, and give her hope.

After 2 days the neurologist, Dr. Ente, examined Judy and looked at the radiology report. Magnetic resonance imaging showed in greater detail just what the CT scan had indicated. He told Don, "There is a blockage there and nothing can be done except wait and see."

A Kafka-esque quality suffuses Don's description of his days and nights at the hospital. He later recalled that apart from evaluations by physical and speech therapists, no doctors visited Judy besides Dr. Ramos, whose exams were routine. When she was awake, Judy often tried to talk but no words came. Don and Annise divined her needs as best they could. Several times a day a nurse would change the IV drip, take Judy's pulse, and make notations on her chart. At night Don found it hard to sleep. Sometimes he wandered the corridors of the 60-bed facility. He came upon the intensive care unit and, looking inside, wondered why Judy was not being cared for there, with its gleaming machines and sophisticated equipment.

Six days after Judy fell down in her kitchen suffering from a stroke, her brain swelling became worse, and on August 28 she was transferred to the much larger Cottage Hospital in Santa Barbara.

Don and Gina were there when she arrived, brought by ambulance. Now a large group of doctors and nurses surrounded her, discussing her case. More images of her brain showed, as the doctors explained, that she was losing one function after another.

"They booted up the MRIs," recalled Don, "and told us she was dead."

In the wake of Judy's death, Don Mead experienced what he recalls as his own serious, albeit temporary, mental decline. Stroke had destroyed his wife's brain and ultimately killed her, and now his own was not working so well. "It seemed like my memory was gone. I could not remember anything. And I didn't know why that happened. But I can tell you, that does happen…. For some reason your brain shuts down. Perhaps it's a self-defense mechanism. I don't know … never understood it. I was not doing well mentally for quite some time."

His family provided support. Both Don's parents were still alive and well, and he had four brothers and a sister. Shortly after Judy's funeral they all went up to the High Sierras, on a camping trip like others they had taken as a family decades before. They stayed at Lake Huntington, near Yosemite, among the dense fir and tall thin pine. "It turned out to be a therapy-rescue thing," Don recalls. At a picnic table they had a grand time eating the Kobe beef that Don and Judy used to market, and though they did not talk about her, he recalls, "Everybody noticed the hole."

Don's decision to ask the people at the hospital about Judy's case, he says, began with benign intentions. He could not put out of his mind the 6 harrowing days. Don later said that he felt the hospital had seemed to lose sight of Judy while she lay paralyzed. The long wait for the neurologist, the fact the MRI machine was not working the first day, and what he viewed as the failure to help her in any way he could perceive—all of it upset him. Too, he had asked about clot-busters but said he had been thoroughly ignored. He said he was never simply and directly informed about either the diagnosis or prognosis—what had happened or what might be expected to happen. Perhaps doctors had done all they could for Judy but he had many questions. With Annise Spangler he discussed it and she too had all sorts of issues.

So in the hope of alerting the hospital to what he perceived as lapses, Don and Annise made an appointment with Linda Everly, Director of

Quality Improvement. But the meeting, which took place a couple of months after Judy's death, did not go well. The Lompoc Community Hospital administration assumed a stance that Don and Annise felt was seemed aggressive and defensive. They talked with Everly and the nurse who had happened to be in the emergency room the morning Don and Judy arrived.

"I am not a combative person, I don't believe," said Don. "I was not going into to do battle with them. I thought I was going in to improve the situation."

Early in the meeting, when Don inquired about tPA, it was only to wonder why she had not received it. He imagined there must be some good reason. Now he was told there was a contraindication: Judy had gotten so dramatically better. Clot-busters were not to be used because of the risk they entailed. "Rapidly improved?" he later recalled. "I was there and she still couldn't move. She still couldn't talk. What rapid improvement?"

The nurse spoke up: "No, your wife—I saw it. She really improved. She regained the use of the right side of her body."

Don recalled being shocked. According to his later testimony, the whole time, from the moment Judy fell down in the kitchen until she died, she could not speak. The whole right side of her body was paralyzed. He saw no improvement. As she lay in the hospital gurney, Judy could work her torso back and forth, and that could draw her leg along with it. At one point a nurse scraped the bottom of Judy's foot and noted a slight twitch. But as far as Don was concerned, this was nothing like improvement, much less recovery.

The conversation with the hospital personnel went nowhere. Don brought a notepad but wrote nothing down. He went away confused and angry. He now believed the hospital was covering up. How or why he could not say, but he knew for certain that when Judy had been moved to a private room at 2 in the afternoon, 5 hours after suffering her stroke, her condition was essentially the same as when they arrived. She never received clot-busters and he never got a good explanation as to why not.

A day or two after that chilly meeting, Don sought legal counsel.

Ten years after FDA approval and one confirmatory study after another, Zivin decided, was long enough. Several NINDS study investigators had already offered expert testimony in cases of alleged malpractice concerning tPA, but he did not. He had acquired experience providing legal testimony, however, in a handful of other cases. Then in 2007 he decided the time had come. He was impressed after a debate in St. Louis, when a doctor in the audience stood up to explain why he did not use tPA: "I work in a little hospital and we just don't have the staffing."

Such excuses were not uncommon, but Zivin said something that provoked a reaction he did not expect. He was blunt and ironic in a way that was extreme even for him: "If you don't have the capability of doing this sort of thing," he replied, "then you should take down the sign at your hospital that says *emergency room.*"

The audience, largely composed of nurses who had learned to use tPA, began to cheer—a sign, he thought, of a shift if not a new readiness. Public awareness of stroke continued to be miserably deficient, and popular knowledge about tPA remained scant. The drug was still the only approved treatment for acute stroke, but the upward trend in using it had progressed from a paltry 1% to perhaps 3%—while theoretically it could be as high as 50%. Meanwhile, much research had been done to show that tPA could be used effectively in the most ordinary hospital settings. At academic medical centers and in the growing number of primary stroke centers, it was considered "standard of care." Yet in several thousand emergency rooms across the United States, it was a treatment more in theory than in fact.

With reluctance—law was not science—Zivin decided to enter what one expert called the "legal quagmire" around tPA. With Bryan A. Liang—a physician, lawyer, and associate professor of health law—he investigated the evolving malpractice record. Legal databases brought up some 33 cases settled or gone to trial. A clear trend emerged: they typically involved failure to provide the drug, not misuse. Database limitations meant the actual number of cases was undoubtedly much higher. Defendants had prevailed about two thirds of the time—no surprise, because malpractice suits typically fail. The success rate for plaintiffs was, in fact, rather on the high side.

In 2008 Zivin published two papers, each aimed at a particular audience and both intended to alert doctors to the changing legal landscape. One of them, written with Liang and biostatistician Robert A. Lew, was published in the *Archives of Neurology.* Another went to the *Annals of Emergency Medicine,* and Zivin was somewhat surprised when it was accepted. But emergency doctors, originally concerned about being sued for using the treatment, were now more worried about litigation for not providing it. "The typical characteristics of a stroke/tPA lawsuit," wrote Zivin and Liang, "is a patient suing an emergency physician who has failed to make or delayed a stroke diagnosis, with the patient not receiving tPA."

Together, the papers combined an overview with data concerning effectiveness. Zivin and his colleagues warned that protection afforded doctors by the limited use of the drug "may not continue in the future." The drug might have once been considered experimental or risky, but this was no longer a durable defense for not giving it. Failure to provide tPA would be increasingly the basis for claims of malpractice, based on evidence that the drug prevents harm.

Because malpractice litigation involves authoritative use of statistical evidence, the article in the *Archives of Neurology* also provided several congruent lines of such analysis, based mainly on the outcomes of the NINDS trials and other studies.

First, a "pooled analysis" including 2,776 patients from all the tPA placebo-controlled trials showed that more than half who were tPA-treated had completely recovered after 3 months. If they received the drug within 2 hours, nearly two thirds *almost* completely recovered; some might get better while suffering from a minor deficit. Similarly, Zivin and colleagues showed that nearly 6 in 10 tPA-treated patients will be either normal or improved at 3 months, with numbers drawn from a re-analysis of the NINDS study data published in 2004 by neurologist Jeffrey Saver (whose work is discussed more completely in Chapter 10).

Finally, a third analysis involved computing all possible comparisons of all patients from the NINDS trials. Using a statistical method designed to measure the differences in scores between populations, tPA- and placebo-treated cases were compared by outcome. The seven-level modified Rankin Scale (mRS; recovery = 0, death = 6) was used to assess patients twice: first when they arrived for emergency treatment and again at 90 days. Raw data from the NINDS study were used for this purpose and, again, the probability that tPA would improve outcome when administered within 3 hours of symptom onset was about 57%.

Zivin foresaw what would happen. Not long after these articles appeared in print, he began receiving inquiries from attorneys, some in search of expert testimony. The numbers in the paper—the robust statistics showing that more than half of the tPA-treated patients recover completely or partly—were of intrinsic interest to malpractice lawyers. In assessing whether harm was done and deciding on damages, many state and local courts use a standard such as a "reasonable degree of medical probability" to help decide whether a patient might have recovered. This is often designated to be "50% plus one patient." Because expert opinions will differ, such a legal formality offers the courts a way to avoid relying on speculation.

Zivin did not relish the prospect of testifying against physicians, but he hoped legal recourse might convince them that failure to treat eligible patients with tPA was itself a decision. Indeed, both in terms of outcome and legal liability, failure to use tPA could outweigh any danger that it might contribute to a bad outcome—such as conversion of an ischemic stroke into a bad hemorrhagic stroke.

One call Zivin received came from Eugene Locken, in Santa Barbara—the lawyer retained by Don Mead. Joined by his stepdaughter Gina, Don brought suit for malpractice. Against everybody, as is usual. They sued Dr. Sadaf Khan, the emergency physician. They included in the suit Dr. Philip Ente, the neurologist with whom Dr. Khan had consulted. Then there was Dr. Maria Cecilia Ramos, the primary care physician assigned to Judy after she was no longer considered an emergency patient. Finally, they sued the Lompoc Valley Medical Center.

Gene Locken, the malpractice attorney in Santa Barbara County who filed the lawsuit on Don and Gina's behalf, believed the case was viable but by no means a slam-dunk. In their favor, the hospital had developed a stroke protocol that included using tPA. Important also was Don's fast reaction in rushing Judy to the emergency room. Locken recalled one tPA stroke case he had pursued, several years earlier, which was settled for a pittance because the patient arrived at the hospital only in the final moments before the therapeutic window closed. Don's contention that he had specifically requested that Judy receive "clot-busters" could also work in his favor.

But there were obstacles, too. Judy's stroke was massive. The NINDS study and other trials indicated only a trend toward more lives saved with tPA (In a 2010 paper, fewer deaths with tPA was in fact shown to reach statistical significance among patients treated within 90 minutes.) At the same time, one could not cogently reason in reverse. One could not conclude from the bare fact of Judy's death that tPA in time would not have rescued or helped her recover, perhaps completely or almost so.

In his deposition, Don recalled Judy: how she was healthy, never smoked or drank more than a glass of wine, always exercised. She was a full partner in his business and after her death he was forced to dramatically cut back the workload. He told about the morning of the stroke and the 6 days after. With chagrin he recalled the hospital staff "not being able to tell me she had a stroke" all through the first day and into the second. When doctors got together as a group to tell him Judy had died, Don said to them: "If I had turned left at the end of the road, instead of right, things would have been different." He meant that, had he driven his white truck not toward Lompoc Valley Medical Center but in the direction of Cottage Hospital, Judy might have survived.

One of the doctors—the "stupid shrink," Don recalled bitterly—replied: "You can't think that way."

As defendants, the doctors who treated Judy Mead answered Gene Locken's questions and defended their decisions. Dr. Khan, the emergency physician, had seen to the patient within moments of her arrival at the hospital. Because Judy was unable to talk, the doctor received a brief medical history from Don; Dr. Khan also took on board information from the nursing staff. Her own notes were incomplete but she wrote that Judy's "left leg would withdraw to pain, the right leg did not move at all to pain." In further notes made that morning, Dr. Khan at one point confused Judy's left and right leg.

The upshot, testified Dr. Khan, was that "certainly a stroke was part of my list of differentials"—that is, one of the diagnoses she considered. In line with hospital protocol governing the use of tPA, she ordered a CT scan. But she also requested a battery of tests, some common and ordinary for a stroke, such as a blood count and electrocardiogram. Others, such as a chest X-ray, were less so.

Judy's loss of language, her facial droop, and weakness on the right side, affecting her arm and face, actually represented a trio of symptoms (in a right-handed person) that physicians regard as proven indications of stroke, based on clinical pathological correlations that have been known for more than one hundred years. The CT scan showed no bleed, so that Judy should have qualified for tPA, and Dr. Khan had taken as much history as she could have needed from Don. If she was really concerned about a hemorrhage in the brain stem, as she testified, the CT scan would be expected to show it; a spinal tap would not be called for. From the symptoms described, there was little reason, as Dr. Khan claimed in her deposition, to seriously consider metabolic syndrome, epileptic seizure, low blood sugar, infection, or brain disease caused by, say, liver dysfunction.

Dr. Khan's failure to provide tPA after the CT scan became the focus of Gene Locken's legal assessment. "What I found in this particular case," said Locken, "led me to believe that the ER physician did not know how to implement the protocol properly." She started down the path to give the drug but he concluded that she did not follow through.

Defending her actions, Dr. Khan made statements that varied dramatically with Don Mead's recollections. She testified that she had informed him about tPA because that was her "custom and practice." But Dr. Khan did not document such a conversation, and Don testified that she did not talk with him about the "clot-busters" he had specifically requested. More substantially, Dr. Khan asserted that tPA was contraindicated because Judy's symptoms were "rapidly improving." She started to be able to move her "right extremity" and some stimuli elicited the word "Ouch." Don testified he had heard something less articulate. The doctor evidently also regarded this as improvement.

Exactly when Dr. Khan decided to consult with a neurologist also came into dispute: in light of her view that Judy was improving, she said, sometime around 11:15 in the morning. The neurologist himself put the time at closer to noon.

Philip Ente recalled in his deposition that he immediately recognized that he was dealing with stroke. But Dr. Khan also told him Judy was "showing spontaneous movement in the right arm and leg," and had said "Ouch" when stimulated.

With Dr. Khan on the phone, Dr. Ente asked her to evaluate Judy's ability to move her right leg.

"I asked her, 'When the leg is up in the air, if you push it down, can she maintain it against your force?' and she said yes. That means the right leg strength had [substantially] improved…."

This interchange was made odd by the fact that Dr. Khan in her notes at one point had confused right and left. If she had also made such an egregious error during her exam while on the phone with Dr. Ente, it might well have affected the recommendation he made. This was never determined, however.

In any case, Dr. Ente advised against tPA. "On initial presentation before CT scan, it was a severe stroke. After she returned from CT scan, I would have called it a rapidly improving, at that point, moderate stroke."

Another reason that he counseled against tPA, he said, was due to his own view of it as a "lethal drug." Citing three articles from the journal *Radiology*, he claimed that, "had we given this patient tPA, statistically there would be a higher chance of her being killed by it."

Now came the experts.

Zivin testified on behalf of Don Mead, with the articles he had just published on the legal situation as key documents. Defense lawyers sought neurologist Gregory W. Albers, director of the stroke center at Stanford University. An imposing figure with a broad smile and high forehead, Albers had proven experience in testifying on behalf of doctors in cases involving tPA. Away from the docket, he and Zivin were on collegial terms and, in fact, had co-authored scientific papers together. Their roles as dueling witnesses was a reminder that law employs science as a rhetorical tool in an adversarial process.

One afternoon in July 2009, the lawyers and Don Mead gathered in Zivin's office for his deposition. After preliminaries, Donald Fesler, Dr. Ente's attorney, questioned him. Zivin explained when, where, and why he thought the neurologist had gone wrong with Judy Mead. He stated that the articles cited by Dr. Ente, the ones the neurologist said he had carefully read and filed away for future reference, were outdated. That is, these articles involved research conducted soon after tPA had been approved in the late 1990s that aimed to discover whether radiological evidence could show whether the drug would be effective in specific types of stroke. The effort, wholly valid at the time, had proved a failure. CT scans have not proved useful in differentiating whether tPA would be effective with any particular patient.

At one point, at Fesler's request Zivin printed out a copy of his CV. The lawyer received the sheaf of papers directly from the printer with a pleasant, "Must be good, it's still warm."

Q. My question to you is: Do any of these publications in
your own CV specifically support any of the opinions
you're going to voice in this case?
A. Yes.
Q. Would you be kind enough just to go through the CV
very quickly and circle the ones that you believe support
your opinions in this case?
A. It would be at least half of them.

During a recess Zivin circled more than 100 publications, beginning with
the first paper that appeared in *Science* in 1985. But it was not just the literature.
Dr. Ente, Zivin testified, had violated the standard of care by not going to the
emergency room himself to examine Judy Mead. Dr. Ente would almost
certainly have performed a more thorough neurological examination than had
Dr. Khan, and that would have cleared up any question of whether Judy was
having a stroke. In Zivin's opinion, Dr. Ente was wrong, too, in recommending
against tPA based on the view that Judy was "rapidly improving." Reliance on
such a sign has become outdated. Stroke symptoms often improve—and they
can also subsequently grow worse. Recent research into outcomes indicated
that tPA should not be withheld based on such signs; no good comes from
waiting once the diagnosis is made.

Zivin then assessed Judy's chances of recovery had she received tPA, based
on his statistical analysis. Nothing as to her individual condition—no risk factor
or stroke type—would change what he could say, positively or negatively, about
her chances. He could predict: 58%, about a 6-in-10 chance for an improved
outcome. The stroke, he agreed, had turned out to be massive—but, he contended, she should have been given the opportunity to recover with tPA.

However, the real failure to treat, Zivin believed, owed not to Dr. Ente but
more directly to Dr. Khan's uncertain appraisal of Judy's symptoms. State law
dictated that as a neurologist, Zivin would not be able to give an opinion as to
whether an emergency physician had made mistakes—Gene Locken had an
emergency physician for that—but he felt there should have been no doubt as
to the diagnosis from the start. The three classic signs—inability to talk, weakness on one side, and facial droop—told the story. Leg movement should not
have been a determining feature; nor should Judy's relatively young age have
interfered. Nothing should have. By symptoms noted and tests ordered, the
doctor had in effect started the process that, if a brain scan did not show a
bleeding stroke, ought to have led to tPA.

Don Mead sat silent through Zivin's deposition, as he had done with all the
other depositions except his own. He had long ago formed his rancher's view of
the emergency room physician who, confronted with Judy, failed to use tPA.

"She was," he recalled thinking, "like a deer in the headlights."

Greg Albers was deposed in late July. Although he testified on behalf of the defendants, Gene Locken elicited testimony that showed in many respects he was in agreement with Zivin. He acknowledged tPA worked, that the results from the NINDS trials were robust. "I don't have any disagreement that approximately 1 out of 3 patients that we treat in general benefit from the therapy."

But he took issue with Zivin in a fundamental, almost philosophical way. While Zivin took the view that predicting the outcome of Judy's stroke was limited to what was known from the randomized studies and the statistical measures, Albers maintained he could say more. Judy's stroke turned out to be particularly severe and so, he thought, it probably would have been fatal in any event. In not giving tPA, in his view, the doctors did no harm because the outcome was predictably bad.

"I don't think tPA would have altered her outcome because I don't think it would be likely to dissolve an internal carotid occlusion. So the answer would be: I don't think she would have survived if she had been treated with t-PA."

Judy's case lay outside the statistics, contended Albers. In malpractice defense, such a strategy is common. "This is what attorneys always get their defense experts to do," said Gene Locken. "Which is to take that particular individual patient out of all of the studies, to make her the exception."

Albers created a plausible account that, to be sure, might persuade a jury. The outcome for any stroke type with tPA is inherently unpredictable on a case-by-case basis, but he offered the claim that "when you mix good prognosis, medium prognosis, and bad prognosis patients.... The good prognosis patients would have higher than 50%, the bad prognosis patients would have considerably lower than 50% good outcome rates." He added, "So based on reasonable medical probability, more likely than not the t-PA would not have opened [Judy's] internal carotid and given her the benefit that one would have hoped for."

The clash of experts—emergency physician experts for both defense and plaintiff also testified—set the table for a resolution. After lawyers heard Zivin's testimony, and took on board both what Albers claimed and also what he conceded, there grew up a general recognition that a settlement was called for. The upshot was an agreement to turn to a professional mediator with a view to settlement.

"Mediation is where you search for common ground to create a resolution," said Gene Locken. The mediator has no power to forge a settlement and does not weigh the facts. He or she seeks to understand the strengths and weaknesses of both plaintiffs and defendants and, ordinarily, plays one against the other.

For Gene Locken on behalf of Don Mead, the mediation took a turn for the better when, after laying out the case on both sides, defense lawyers challenged him on the percentages. Zivin had testified for stroke and tPA, to be sure—but what about Judy's middle cerebral artery stroke? Zivin had not testified to that and Albers had used it as an escape hatch. "You're going to have to show us some article that supports what you're contending," they told him.

Locken had come to mediation prepared. A small study that used magnetic resonance imaging, published in *Stroke* in 2008, showed that patients with middle cerebral artery stroke can improve with tPA. There were only 14 patients, but the results, with 57% of patients having a favorable outcome, passed the 50-plus percent test and satisfied the threshold in California. All parties moved toward a resolution, or settlement, the terms of which, it was agreed, were not to be publicly disclosed.

From the case of Judy Mead, interested parties could draw useful lessons about how to behave—not just to avoid lawsuits but to do the right thing. Individual physicians could acknowledge that acute stroke is a treatable condition and learn how and when to use tPA. Hospital administrators could ensure that all personnel connected with emergency treatment for stroke be fully current and up to date on thrombolysis. The size of their institution should not be a factor, nor should local conditions afford cover for failure to treat acute ischemic stroke. If a service cannot meet that standard, it should arrange for patients to bypass their hospital and go directly to others that are prepared to treat strokes as the emergencies they truly are.

But for individuals, for all potential stroke victims and their families and friends, the learning curve is stark yet terribly ambiguous. For them the question Don Mead posed to the doctors the moment they declared his wife was dead represents the greatest lesson from litigation concerning tPA. Any expectation of emergency care is compromised in case of stroke. Unless one lives next door to a primary stroke center, what assurance may we have of being properly evaluated and treated? How do we know beforehand whether the closest hospital has a trained staff and follows a stroke protocol and uses tPA?

The answer is: Mostly, we have no assurance. We do not know.

Although not advanced in acute stroke therapy, Chinese researchers conducted their own clinical research and several times invited Zivin to China to keep them current with what was happening in the United States and elsewhere. While visiting in 1998, at one point he could only stand aside as a group of investigators, in front of a series of brain images, held a lively, even vociferous discussion. They talked too fast for his translator to keep up but one had to admire their level of engagement.

One of them suddenly turned to Zivin. He was a high-level physician, dressed in a dark green military uniform. Grimly, he pronounced: "You NIH guys could never have treated patients as fast as you said you did."

Zivin looked at the doctor, took notice of the gleaming revolver holstered across his chest, and said: "You're right."

Today, countries throughout the world are contending with the use of tPA for stroke, each in its own way and according to various factors that affect the adoption of any treatment. China, still underdeveloped by the standards of Western medicine, struggles with its level of care, complex geography, and the cost of thrombolysis. Across the globe, broad outlines are similar. Traditional ingrained beliefs and widespread lack of knowledge about stroke remain stubbornly entrenched, if not as pervasive as in the past. Numbers of tPA-treated patients in some countries are rising substantially, with several now matching or exceeding the best academic centers in the United States. Although national health care systems ensure a measure of uniformity, centralization with only a small number of well-equipped hospitals makes it difficult to provide acute care fast to many patients. Wealth and regional variation also play a role. Emergency care for stroke, in short, depends upon functioning health care systems able to embrace and use tPA. Countries in which thrombolysis is essentially not to be had—the no-shows—include the poorest nations in the developing world, which lack resources to treat not just stroke but most diseases. But a number of countries in the first world, including England and Japan, are latecomers for idiosyncratic reasons of their own.

For the European Union, approval of tPA for stroke came only in 2002 and provisionally, with requirements for an international monitoring study and another randomized trial, both of which turned out in its favor by 2007 and 2008, respectively (the observational Safety Implementation Thrombolysis in Stroke–Monitoring Study [SITS–MOST] and the third incarnation of the European Cooperative Acute Stroke Study [ECASS-III]). Issues of infrastructure for emergency treatment and public awareness were new to many countries, though not all. "There is a long way to go before most stroke patients have a fair likelihood of receiving good care," according to Markku Kaste, a neurologist long associated with tPA and one of the organizers of the ECASS series of trials.

Doctors in Finland, where Kaste is based, treat more patients per million strokes with thrombolysis than any other country in Europe. With a relatively homogeneous population of about 5 million, Finland also benefits from geography—the country is small and flat—and a centralized hospital system. Kaste and colleagues made a determined effort to reorganize emergency stroke care beginning in the late 1990s.

Elsewhere, throughout most of Europe, thrombolysis for stroke is an evolving work in progress. Didier Leys, from his hospital perch in the old city of Lille, northernmost France, ponders the European map. A neurologist at Hôpital Roger Salengro, a large university medical center, Leys is former head of the French Stroke Society and currently chairs the European Stroke Organization.

"We cannot give tPA in France if we are not in a stroke unit," he points out. "This is a legal issue."

Nevertheless, France has moved forward since 2002. Government-led reforms in 2003 and 2007 sought to improve organization of care and to establish dedicated stroke units in smaller hospitals. Some places lack emergency rooms and CT scanners, making availability of acute stroke treatment a problem. The emergency medical service—"Call 15," the equivalent of "Call 911"—is being successfully enlisted to organize patient transportation to the nearest stroke center. Use of tPA has advanced accordingly, with some large hospitals, by 2008, treating more than 100 patients annually and smaller centers, more than 50. This represents about a five-fold increase in just 3 years.

"Which is not bad," says Leys. "It's really an improvement."

Encouraging, too, he says, is that patients are arriving earlier. The success of ECASS III and repeated regional public information campaigns have helped to achieve greater penetration in the population as a whole, though it is still far from optimal.

Other countries in the 22-member European Union present a mixed picture.

"In Italy it is dependent on where you are," continues Leys. "In Milan or Rome, for example, you have very high-level units; but in other parts, it is seriously deficient. You have the best and the worst." In the Netherlands, as in many other European countries, acute stroke care is rather centralized in a few hospitals. In Belgium, like Italy, location is important, with disparities according to region.

"Spain is working well," says Didier, with excellent centers in major population centers such as Barcelona and Madrid. "Portugal is a little bit more difficult."

Eastern Europe, where rates of stroke are thought to be higher that in Mediterranean countries, shows patchwork success. Effective use of tPA in several former Soviet-bloc countries, especially Hungary but also Poland, is notable but not the norm. "If you go more to the eastern part of Europe, the former Soviet Union, the Ukraine and so on," says Leys, "it's another world." With the importance of rapid transport and CT scan, defective health care systems defeat the use of tPA.

To suggest tPA got off on the wrong foot in the United Kingdom is more than an understatement. The "battle of the clot-busters" predates its use with stroke. As we discussed in Chapter 6, when large trials compared tPA with streptokinase for heart attack, the older and less expensive drug performed quite well. In 1991, British doctors felt seriously snubbed when a famous American cardiologist, Burton Sobel, ignored their data favoring streptokinase and extolled tPA—and some suspected this was due to financial gains he stood to make from Genentech stock options. At a conference, British cardiovascular expert Peter Sleight responded with the eccentricity considered typical for an Oxford professor. Removing his shoes and socks, he padded onstage to tell a huge audience—this took place in a cavernous auditorium in Atlanta, Georgia— that he was a visiting "barefoot doctor." His sarcasm underscored disdain for the newer, more costly drug; it seems to have become entrenched in British medical culture.

Streptokinase went on to become the drug of choice in England for heart attack. Consequently, British physicians—not necessarily neurologists, who were not commonly involved in emergency stroke care—were reluctant to accept results of the NINDS trials or to use tPA. It was as if they believed strep-tokinase *ought* to work as well with stroke—even as trials with that drug were repeatedly shut down before completion because of excess harm due to hemor-rhage. Objections to the NINDS study were persistently voiced by some in the United Kingdom on a variety of counts. A marked preference for large trials with thousands of patients was one factor; by such a standard the NINDS study seemed small. "There is still relatively poor evidence for the use of thrombolysis in acute ischemic stroke, nothing like as good evidence for myocardial infarc-tion," asserted Charles Warlow, a distinguished neurologist with the University of Edinburgh, in 2009. He pointed to just several thousand patients in all the randomized tPA trials for stroke trials as compared with upwards of 60,000 for heart attack. He also voiced an old claim that randomization in the NINDS trial was defective. He and colleagues currently run the long-running International Stroke Trial (IST-III), which has, however, advanced toward completion rather slowly.

Indeed, a full explanation of the science and politics around tPA and medi-cine in the U.K. probably requires a book of its own. Kennedy Lees, a professor of cerebrovascular medicine at the University of Glasgow, in Scotland, was using tPA on an off-label basis prior to approval and has since developed a highly proactive program where use of thrombolysis appears to dwarf that at nearby Edinburgh. He is highly critical of the slow adoption of tPA in the U.K. and believes that it was inappropriate to be "creating uncertainty" in the wake of the NINDS study. The negative reaction arose from genuine doubt whether the drug could safely be used in practice. But, he adds, "Some of it was doubt created by listening to those who had a very good way with words and could spin the data very well."

In 2005 neurologist Alastair Buchan returned to England, where he found the situation retarded there "by about 10 to 15 years." While himself a British physician out of Oxford, Buchan himself was an exception: he had also trained in the United States, where he worked on early tPA studies, and in Canada. There he became an instrumental figure in gaining conditional endorsement for tPA in 1999 and, after a safety and efficacy trial, full approval 2 years later. At Foothills Hospital, which serves all of Calgary, he achieved high rates of tPA use—sometimes as high as 15%—and other regions fared similarly. With neu-rologists treating emergencies and on call day and night, Buchan maintains, "The Canadian system has sort of a much better system of open access than perhaps any privatized system, which you have in the States."

Although Buchan hoped to replicate some of the success he had in Canada, England's long lag has led to systemic backwardness. A recent report from the

Stroke Association describes chronic delays in diagnosis, serious problems with misdiagnosis, ineffectiveness of ambulance services, and deficient expertise in radiology. To remedy the situation, the National Health Service has developed a strategy and campaign launched in February 2009 that included nationwide television advertising—unknown in the United States. The British public is now being urged to "Act F.A.S.T.—Facial weakness, Arm weakness, Speech problems, Time to call 999 for an ambulance…" But widespread public education concerning thrombolysis and tPA remains very much a work in progress.

In Germany the case was quite different: enthusiasm for tPA among physicians is due in large part to clinical research on thrombolysis with its own partly distinct history (Genentech licensed alteplase [tPA] to the Germany-based Boehringer Ingelheim, which distributes it in Europe as Actylase). In addition, for neurologists to treat acute stroke is the rule rather than the exception, and this has been the case for 50 years. Most prominent among them is Werner Hacke, chairman of the Department of Neurology at the University of Heidelberg. Hacke, who collects Harley-Davidson motorcycles and listens to heavy metal rock, self-consciously does not fit the mold of the office-based neurologist. He is quick to point to recent advances on the continent, with roots in the past: "It all started in Europe, and we use [tPA] much more than you guys in the States."

Hacke delivered the first reports of thrombolysis for stroke, using streptokinase or urokinase, in 1981. Other studies emerged from Germany over the next two decades; a majority of patients in the first two incarnations of ECASS were recruited there. The ECASS series, which Hacke helped lead, represents a touchstone for tPA with both general encouragement and regulatory repercussions. From a European point of view, ECASS III in particular constituted an independent confirmation of the NINDS study.

The numbers in Germany attest to success not yet found elsewhere in Europe. For the acute stroke program started 15 years ago, and some 235 acute stroke care units serve 80 million Germans. Hacke's own relatively prosperous state, Baden-Württemberg, is home to 10 million inhabitants, for which there are 42 stroke units. In 2008, 8% of all stroke patients in the state received tPA—including all ages and hemorrhagic strokes; the figure was as high as 20% in selected centers. Although similar percentages exist in the most active centers in the United States, he adds, "You don't have it on a population-wide pattern."

That Japan became a latecomer to tPA for stroke seems ironic because researchers there were at the forefront of early efforts to test thrombolytics for stroke. Some of the earliest trials during the 1990s used an almost identical drug, duteplase, with a 6-hour window, and showed promising results. But trials with that drug ended after Genentech prevailed in a patent dispute with

Burroughs Wellcome. Meanwhile, after the NINDS study, concern about the especially high rates of mortality of stroke in the Japanese population—a long-standing conundrum—made confirmatory testing a crucial issue. But the state of stroke management in Japan, generally speaking, remained unclear until Takenori Yamaguchi led a nationwide study in 1999. Finally, the Japan Alteplase Clinical Trial (J-ACT), an open-label trial conducted in 2002 with a somewhat reduced dosage, provided positive data. The long-delayed result was that tPA was approved for stroke in late 2005, and subsequent monitoring studies have shown the familiar rates of success.

Implementation of acute stroke care in Japan must contend with geography, because populations in both mountainous regions and outlying islands are difficult to serve. Similarly, the familiar problem of public awareness is as acute among the Japanese as elsewhere, according to Yamaguchi; he suggests it may be improved through legislation.

In spite of the kind of success seen in Germany, Austria, and Finland, no country in the world has achieved what could be regarded as a practical upper limit; that number is not known. Just as many heart attack patients do not reach the emergency room even today, delays of all kinds will always mean many stroke patients will not be eligible for tPA. Although time-to-treatment will remain a significant barrier, it also provides an opportunity on which to build universal recognition of the signs and symptoms of stroke and to convey the knowledge that time is brain and treatment can be had.

Finally, the use of tPA should be understood within the larger context of a global epidemic. Worldwide, the human cost and economic burden of stroke are enormous, with permanent disability affecting an estimated 5 million people every year. The focus here has been on relatively well-off countries in which genuine emergency care, and hence tPA, are available, but that is not to ignore prospects for treating acute stroke once a threshold of prosperity makes possible advanced interventions. For the present and immediate future, public health measures for poor and developing countries will be largely limited to a focus on prevention, to efforts to address risk factors, and the use of antihypertensive medications. But the tragically high numbers of permanently disabled stroke victims in these countries should be a stark reminder of the magnitude of damage that stroke inflicts and of the corresponding prospects for both prevention and treatment.

*T*oday clear choices confront physicians and hospitals—while patients have yet to benefit in anything approaching adequate numbers. Fifteen years after tPA was approved for stroke in the United States, the means are at hand for the drug to be widely adopted and thoroughly integrated as the standard of care, as customary and accepted practice. Primary care doctors of all stripes should be trained well enough to administer it, much as they are able to treat heart attack in an emergency. In the awkward, trademarked jargon of the American Heart Association, hospitals and medical centers should "Get With the Guidelines" and build infrastructure, create protocols, and train staff. But more, *everyone*— potential stroke victims, their families, friends, and bystanders—should be aware of the major symptoms of stroke and be prepared to see them as signs of an acute emergency with a ticking clock. They should know about tPA—that treatment is available if they react fast, that time is brain.

This book began with Julie Milanese, the young San Franciscan who, one late afternoon in 2004, suffered a stroke. The knowledge and awareness of people around her ensured that she was rushed to the hospital. There she received tPA. When her family left her that night, she was paralyzed on one side of her body; her speech was slurred and her thinking affected. Doctors assessed her with a score of 11 on the National Institutes of Health Stroke Scale, which is borderline severe. Theoretically, any outcome was possible. She could be expected to improve a little or a lot, or recover completely. She might further decline, then stabilize at some level of disability; or she could sustain yet another stroke and die. Seemingly spontaneous recoveries from stroke do occur, but for Julie that prospect, by 8 o'clock that evening, was long past.

Julie's family and her fiancé, Doug, spent a night desperate with worry. Her mother was all the more distraught because her own mother, Mary, had been confined for the past 15 years to a wheelchair, stroke-paralyzed, cared for in a nursing home.

The next morning, when they returned to the hospital, they found Julie trying to eat breakfast with her left hand. She recovered clarity of thought, speech, and movement over the next several days. She remained hospitalized for a heart operation to correct a congenital condition known as a patent foramen ovale. Best described as a hole in the septum that divides the atrial chambers of the heart, her doctors held it responsible—and it might have been, or not—for transmitting to the arterial system, thence to the brain, the venous clot that caused her stroke.

Julie checked out of the UCSF Medical Center 10 days later, on October 9, 2004: "I came to the hospital completely paralyzed on my left side. I left speaking clearly and walked out. I was cleared of all physical and occupational therapy."

The ordeal left her fatigued. Although she could use it without difficulty, her left arm felt strange; in the ensuing weeks and months she exercised to reconnect and reintegrate it. Serious as ever, she took time off from work while continuing to plan for her marriage. As Doug, her fiancé, well understood, Julie represented "the best-case scenario of what can happen between recognition of a stroke, treatment, and the results afterward."

But Julie was one of a lucky few: just over 1% of all ischemic stroke victims received tPA between 1998 and 2004, the year she had her stroke. Those numbers would improve a little over the next 4 years, and today in the United States an estimated 3% to 8% of acute stroke patients receive tPA—although nobody knows the exact number. In brief, even if victims suffer a stroke and reach a hospital in minutes, their chances of receiving the drug are at best hit or miss— depending on where they live, what emergency room they land in, which doctor treats them. Although the numbers have been improving, about three quarters of hospitals in the United States have not yet instituted the protocol recommended by the Joint Commission, an organization that runs accreditation programs for health care organizations.

Blame for such meager results could be spread wide if one sought to fault the stakeholders. The American Heart Association had endorsed tPA for stroke soon after the FDA approved it, and it made subsequent efforts to improve the organization of stroke care. But in the realm of public education it made only feeble efforts to reach what it considers its core constituency: the general public. In cooperation with the Ad Council, which creates public service advertising, it created a series of shock advertisements that are broadcast hardly anywhere. Such fund-raising mechanisms as telethons or golf tournaments have never happened. Especially when Medicare reimbursement was wholly inadequate, the large insurance companies might have noted that the drug is cost-effective, but they did nothing to expand its use. Even without short-term profitability Genentech might have advertised with greater enthusiasm; instead it stayed largely on the sidelines. In brief, by comparison with heart attack or cancer, little was spent to enhance public awareness. Before tPA, stroke was long ignored. Afterwards, its advent only underscored how the old pessimism had a long reach into both psyche and pocketbook.

But more productive than recrimination is to understand that the core difficulty today consists in moving tPA from the realm of scientific medicine into the more diffuse and unruly arena of health care. New treatments of all kinds invariably face issues of acceptance and adoption by doctors, who on the whole are conservative by nature and cautious by training. With tPA for stroke, long-running controversy and the tenacity of doubt have inhibited efforts to raise widespread awareness. The tragedy is that such doubt, originally part of normal science and medicine, created such high barriers. In emergency medicine especially, over-dependency on epidemiology at the expense of the underlying science meant that the drug's dangers were exaggerated and its efficacy minimized. The best to be said: historic and game-changing innovations in medicine have often enough faced similar negative forces—examples include vaccination, antisepsis, and the treatment of heart attack. In this sense, tPA for stroke is arguably one of the most controversial drug treatments ever approved and brought to market.

"A lot of people all thought that they were doing the right thing, and as a consequence hundreds of thousands if not millions of people were unnecessarily damaged." With those words, Justin Zivin introduced himself to John Simmons during their first substantial conversation, by telephone, in early February 2007. Months would pass before they met face to face. Zivin had been considering writing a book about tPA and stroke for several years. His main aim, he explained, was to widely disseminate knowledge about the only available treatment for a common, crippling, and life-destroying disorder—a drug approved by the FDA, widely endorsed yet vastly underused. In addition, he wanted to tell some of his own story because he had played a significant role in developing tPA for stroke and he was angry about some of what happened. He wanted to write a book that would explain and help rectify the mistakes he believed had helped create and prolong the controversy surrounding the drug, and he was seeking a collaborator. He acknowledged considerable frustration, but that was not the point: the goal was the practical one of raising awareness.

Simmons wrote both about the history of science and medicine and about contemporary issues in medicine, but he did not typically look into controversies unless they were old. Among many others, he had sketched the agonies of Ignaz Semmelweis, who was famously ignored after he showed that childbed fever was due to the unclean hands of doctors themselves; he had discussed arguments over vaccination between Robert Koch and Louis Pasteur. By the time Simmons described the famous dispute over discovery of the human immunodeficiency virus (HIV) by Robert Gallo and Luc Montagnier, the headlines were long past. He always tried to bring these stories down to earth; time had usually detoxified them and made real people of heroes. Did tPA for stroke belong with these historic disputes around discoveries by the embattled and vindicated? Simmons initially doubted it: few stories about a single drug warrant book-length treatment.

But the drug proved to be everything Zivin claimed for it. By general agreement it was the most contentious drug ever used in neurology. Even after seemingly endless debates in journals and conferences had ended in widespread acknowledgment that tPA worked, there remained a hard core of pessimists and naysayers. Although recommended by a host of professional and nonprofit organizations, reluctance in emergency medicine still amounted to a roadblock at the point of care. Many emergency physicians were rooted in a defensive posture, stuck there by rejection embedded in their culture. And by no means was it clear that recent findings, which clarified the benefits and risks of tPA, had fully penetrated even the neurological community. At the same time, and most importantly, the public remained unenlightened and oblivious. In 2009 people were ignorant about stroke in the same way that a half century ago everybody knew next to nothing about heart attack.

Simplicity—*know the symptoms, call 911*—did not disturb the persistent somnolence around tPA. In New York in June 2008, Zivin met with Simmons, and they talked all day. At one point, from his office Simmons telephoned a local hospital, a proverbial stone's throw from his home on Staten Island. He wanted to know: if he was having a stroke right now, did the hospital have a stroke center? Good question. He was transferred to emergency services. The extension buzzed and he waited. "The clock is ticking," observed Zivin. Several moments passed. Finally a helpful woman picked up. To the question: "If I'm having a stroke, do you have a stroke center?" she did not have an answer. She went away. "Three minutes," said Zivin as they waited. Eventually she came back on the line.

"We don't have a neurologist in house," she said. "You have to call your neurologist. You call and he comes."

"Thank you very much."

"Have I made my point?" asked Zivin.

To be sure, the situation by 2007 was not as grim or perplexing as it had been in the first several years after FDA approval. The advent of tPA, even though controversial, provoked unprecedented interest in acute stroke. The concept of the primary stroke center came of age in about 2000, and such centers were being established at a growing number of hospitals and medical centers. It generated special interest and action in academic and teaching institutions and gradually reached some smaller hospitals as well, both urban and rural. But the hostility of many emergency physicians, continuing indifference among neurologists, and ignorance on the part of primary care doctors left whole communities underserved and most people, a huge majority, uninformed about either tPA or stroke.

The surprising thing about tPA, in terms of research, was that it turned out to be both a scientific breakthrough and one of a kind. For several years it helped accelerate a search for drugs to further protect the brain during stroke. Drug companies sought agents to keep ischemic tissue alive and lengthen the treatment window. A host of substances showed promise in animals, mainly rats, as researchers targeted the various chemical pathways involved in the destructive insults to the brain during stroke. But when moved into clinical trials, the promising drugs all failed. To date, efforts to discover a new and better form of tPA have also been unsuccessful.

So unexpected seemed the washout of an entire prospective generation of "neuroprotectives" that academic neurologists could scarcely get over it: how could so many trials go wrong? One article in the journal *Stroke* identified no less than nine "pitfalls" to which researchers had fallen victim. Perhaps the most conspicuous mistake was that pharmaceutical companies sought a drug with a time-to-treatment window longer than 3 hours. Future trial design would need to respect the dictum that time is brain. In 2006, a review by Jeff Saver, a neurologist at UCLA, sought and found in the literature a consensus about the ramp-up of damage during a stroke: 1.9 million neurons lost *each minute*, with collateral destruction of 14 billion synapses.

Then, too, surprise at so many failures was due to the success of tPA. New cancer drugs, for example, disappoint with great regularity but, due to high levels of funding and the war mentality associated with the disease, the pipeline never dries up; new candidates are always in trials. But drug companies largely abandoned the search for neuroprotectives. Sentiment among academic neurologists held that it would take a new generation of drug company executives to reignite interest in stroke drugs to save the brain. There remained tPA.

Something of a personal nature attracted Simmons to stroke and to collaboration with Zivin on a book about tPA. The death at 82 of his father, Lou, in the wake of an ischemic stroke, remained embedded in his memory; he still felt aggrieved and angry because the cardiologist had wanted to keep him alive no matter how severe the damage.

"He has a massive infarct," said the doctor, who recommended and indeed was planning to install a pacemaker in Lou's heart so he could be sent home by ambulance to spend the final months of his life in a hospital bed, spoon-fed and without language. "It's a simple procedure."

But also something Lou never would have wanted. Born in 1898, the year of the Spanish-American War, he had survived a ruptured appendix at age 40 to father a second son at age 51. He lived through two heart attacks in an era where nothing could be done but adhere to a bland diet and hope for the best; then he lost a kidney to stones. Arthritis gnarled his fingers, his arteries hardened, his prostate enlarged. But his mind was sharp and, as he puffed on one of his 33 unfiltered cigarettes each day and sipped Scotch over ice, he told anyone who would listen that he did not want to linger before death, bedridden or mentally impaired.

Simmons and his brother, Garner, prevailed on the cardiologist at St. John's Hospital in Santa Monica: no pacemaker. Later, though, Garner recalled how the doctor continued to behave churlishly, retailing guilt while their father was in a coma. Lou never spoke another word nor walked a step before he died a couple of months later.

A curious repercussion to all this, which took place in 1981, was that Simmons recalled reading Zivin's first article in *Science* several years later. He did not clip it, as he did some articles at the time, but he remembered the rabbits and some molecule about which he knew nothing. He wondered vaguely about a connection without being sure when, about a decade later, he heard there was a treatment for stroke. Only in meeting Zivin did he learn about tPA and the controversies surrounding it.

Those disputes clearly constrained public awareness and obscured better news. Statistics from the NINDS study, endlessly repeated in literally thousands of articles in medical journals and the popular press, were good numbers, but they told only part of the story: a revision based on a more detailed analysis shows tPA to be still more effective and less likely to cause harm than the original statistics suggested.

Even in 1996 the widely divergent reactions among physicians were cause for perplexity; in retrospect, they are revealing. Zivin, who had worked in the laboratory with tPA nearly from the beginning and knew its potency, was surprised when the NINDS study was not halted with fewer than the planned 300 patients. At the other end of the spectrum were the British researchers who thought that thousands of patients ought to have been randomized. In one early evaluation, Swiss stroke expert Julien Bogousslavsky described the risk-to-benefit ratio as "narrow" even though the absolute benefit he cited (12%) was by most standards huge. Long after it became clear that no one was going to risk patients' health with more tPA-versus-placebo randomized trials with a 3-hour time window, physicians whose skepticism ranged from mild to denunciatory continued to call for them. If one part of the problem was that most doctors are uncomfortable with statistics, another must be the numbers themselves.

A couple of years after the NINDS study, Jeff Saver began to question whether he or anybody really understood the results. Carefully designed by a group of biostatisticians who discussed the various measures in a special workshop, the results had been purposely framed in conservative terms in order not to oversell the treatment benefit. If they seemed clear enough to NINDS investigators—and they certainly showed tPA was effective—critics nevertheless succeeded in questioning the drug's effectiveness. Why was that?

"The treatment effect must be huge if we detected it in such a small trial," reasoned Saver. "But the way we're describing the treatment effect, it doesn't seem that big. So it must be that we were not describing it in the right way."

Indeed, two particular numbers to emerge from the NINDS study gave pause—not because they were wrong, but rather, incomplete. These were the "number needed to treat" (NNT) and "number needed to harm" (NNH). In recent years the NNT has become a useful way to help doctors decide whether an individual patient should receive a treatment based on risks and benefits as revealed by randomized trials. Similarly, the NNH can help gauge potential danger. Developed only in the late 1980s, the concepts of NNT and NNH are relatively new; most doctors practicing today did not learn them in medical school. On average, for example, antibiotics need to be used on 16 dog bites before one case of infection is prevented. Similarly, give aspirin to 102 patients for 1 year, and there will be one stroke less.

For tPA the NNT based on the NINDS study was 8.4—quite comparable with the best treatments, especially in view of the severity of the disease. Some physicians did not fully understand the concept or else did not read the original study. They took the number literally and believed that statistically it meant about one patient in eight would be helped, while seven of eight would not be helped. In addition, skeptics liked to take this number as a negative. The NINDS study, wrote Robert C. Solomon, "yields a number needed to treat of 9 and a number needed to harm of 17—numbers that hardly support a statement that the therapy is 'highly efficacious.'" Solomon then used this assertion as a bludgeon to denigrate the entire study, continuing with spleen: "All of the other numbers that seem positive are the product of statistical manipulations and data snooping in an effort to demonstrate benefit by post-hoc analysis of unplanned subgroups, methods that are well understood to be useful only to generate hypotheses to test in further prospective RCTs."

In fact, the NNT was highly conservative and the NNH was actually much greater than 17. As Jeff Saver noticed, the NINDS statisticians had framed their results in terms of "dichotomized endpoints." Only patients who enjoyed full or almost complete recovery were considered to have a positive outcome; those with every other result—from disabled-but-able-to-walk to death—were considered to have a negative outcome. This method had the advantage of clarity but came at a price. Using the 42-point NIH Stroke Scale, for example, a score of 0 or 1 put patients in the positive camp; every other score, from 2 to 42, was counted as negative. It did not matter whether a patient was dead or alive and completely independent yet unable to return to work; the outcome was counted as negative in both cases.

"That type of dichotomization was standard in the field at the time," said Saver, "and it grew out of the fact that many of the initial clinical trials were done with conditions that had intrinsic binary endpoints." With either heart attack or cancer, for example, only survival really matters. But stroke is both a lethal and a crippling disease, and the damage it inflicts is of varied severity. "What statisticians will tell you is that whenever you dichotomize information, you wind up throwing out information. And you're reducing the power of your trial."

Using statistical tools developed after the NINDS study was published, Saver recalculated. He created a virtual model of 100 patients that reflected the percentage outcomes from the NINDS trials according to the modified Rankin Scale (mRS)—the simple seven-level appraisal tool that determines how a patient ends up, ranging from perfectly well (0) to dead (6). He then asked experts—neurologists and emergency physicians—to suggest how the individual outcomes of tPA- and placebo-treated patients might be distributed based on the overall percentages in conformity with the NINDS results.

Results from this exercise provided new numbers for help and harm. "The NNT for 1 additional patient to have a better outcome by 1 or more grades than he or she would have had with placebo," wrote Saver, "was 3.1." In other words, treat three patients and help one of them. Similarly, at least 30 patients needed to be treated to harm one; this figure, depending on whether serious disability and death are combined, could range as high as 1 in 100.

The 2009 International Stroke Conference took place in San Diego, where Zivin still lived and worked; and as this book took shape, his co-author attended.

As a journalist, sometimes as a medical writer-analyst, Simmons had covered any number of medical meetings—but never stroke. The annual conference is modest relative to oncology and cardiology—and so disproportionately small in terms of the overall morbidity and mortality that stroke inflicts. It attracts several thousand stroke experts and neurologists, together with neurosurgeons, emergency medicine physicians, biostatisticians, nurses, and anyone clinically connected with stroke. Like most conferences, it is 3 days of men and women gathering in small groups and flowing into high-ceilinged darkened halls to sit before stages with podiums and tables lined with suited specialist-experts in front of wide screens that show PowerPoint presentations. But these meetings are also socially and scientifically interactive. Zivin typically spends most of his time in the halls outside the big rooms, talking with colleagues.

Change and even transformation were on display at Stroke 2009. The conference has come to reflect a growing emphasis on epidemiology and science. In the 1980s, when Zivin first began attending, the meeting was not really interesting. Basic scientists avoided it—still do—so there was little enough biochemistry or molecular biology; rather, physicians and surgeons would talk about their collections of intriguing cases and rare disorders. The gray eminences at the time—C. Miller Fischer, Fred Plum, Clark Millikan, and others—had crafted their reputations by investigating stroke and creating new classifications and subtypes of brain disease. When they rose to speak, attendees listened with reverence. But in point of fact most papers were largely confined to description and taxonomy: nothing could be done for acute stroke patients, truth to tell, nor help much afterward. Into the 1980s the best that neurology had to offer was the anticoagulant heparin—and no one really knew if it worked.

But genuine advances for acute stroke were nevertheless on the horizon prior to tPA. Computerized tomography revolutionized X-rays of the brain in the 1970s, while several large studies, about the same time, brought to bear serious epidemiology. A pioneering randomized trial showed that patients with clogged carotid arteries might avoid stroke by undergoing surgery. Another famous trial, led by Canadian neurologist Henry Barnett, showed that aspirin could help prevent stroke. As the complexion of research changed, so did the temperaments of its leading figures. James T. Robertson has recalled the arrival of a generation of neurologists and neurosurgeons "with uncommon zeal for achievement and a rabidly competitive nature."

Skepticism greeted Zivin when he first experimented with tPA and exposed his research at the International Stroke Conference. His statistical approach, his rabbits, and this bioengineered clot-buster that the cardiologists were toying with—none of this met with warm embrace. He recalled how, in 1986, standing in front of his poster, Mark L. Dyken, a well-known stroke doctor and author of textbooks, stopped to read it. He said, shaking his head with a small laugh, alluding to the streptokinase trials of the previous decade: "Oh, we tried thrombolysis years ago and it didn't work."

But a quarter century later, at Stroke 2009, thrombolysis did work and tPA, still the only proven and approved treatment, was a dominant theme. A number of the original NINDS study investigators could be seen among the throng at the San Diego Convention Center, themselves now on the road to gray eminence. Some gave talks: John Marler and Joe Broderick on the time window to treatment; Jim Grotta on chilling the stroked brain to save it—a strategy that seems to be working for a select few victims. The role the NINDS study had played in most of their careers was by no means negligible.

Not NINDS but the recent success of ECASS III, the international randomized control trial that extended the treatment window to 4.5 hours, represented the most talked-about boon for tPA. The American Heart Association was soon to change its guidelines to reflect as much, just like the Europeans had done; so too the Canadians. Werner Hacke, who had led the study, was on hand to parse the results.

"We don't have to go into detail," the German neurologist told the packed audience while showing a comparison of tPA with placebo that needed no interpretation. "It's pretty obvious that [tPA] is positive over the whole spectrum of modified Rankin shift analysis."

A former skeptic from England, Peter Sandercock, explained that his ongoing trial, known as International Stroke Trial (IST-3), could be expected to demonstrate more specifics about which subgroups of patients would benefit. A tendency to not give tPA to people over 80 years old might well prove unjustified. "Your chances of getting tPA in an American hospital are vanishingly small the nearer you get to 90 years," said Sandercock. Of several thousand patients in all the randomized control trials to date, only 42 have been octogenarians.

When a treatment works and is not too difficult to administer, physicians usually find a way. Edward Jenner discovered his vaccine for smallpox a century before refrigeration, which meant it had to be fabricated directly from the pustules of victims. Teenage boys who had not been immunized were recruited as reservoirs for the vaccine and made mildly sick as they were transported to distant lands aboard ships that sailed the world. Although tPA for stroke required nothing so drastic, the problem of fast diagnosis and timely delivery was stubborn.

One consequence at Stroke 2009 was a lively and engaging debate that pitted the telephone against computerized televised consultations. Which of them, when a question arose, was best for a fast and accurate decision whether to treat with tPA? Although advice by phone can lead to the right choice much of the time, the remote neurologist relies on verbal description, the radiology report, and whatever information blood tests provide. With telemedicine, by contrast, the remote neurologist actually sees, communicates with, and evaluates the patient.

Nancy Edwards, an emergency physician and director of the stroke program at the small Tobey Hospital in Wareham, Massachusetts, made an impressive case for telemedicine. With no local neurologist to call, she gave tPA only about once a year; other patients might be shipped off to larger medical centers. But now stroke victims, via audio and visual feed, could be brought before doctors located at Massachusetts General Hospital. The initial work and expense of installing equipment and training staff was repaid by enhanced confidence in diagnosis and satisfaction among patients.

"We used to give tPA one or two times a year when we were just a stand-alone ED doing it," said Edwards. "But in the first 18 months after we started telestroke and were designated as a primary stroke center, we gave tPA ten times."

But James L. Frey, chief of the neurovascular section at Barrow Neurological Institute in Phoenix, Arizona, was having none of telemedicine. The phone is good enough, he asserted, simple and fast. *Lancet Neurology* had published an article comparing the two methods in 2008. Maybe telemedicine had an edge in diagnosis, but with the telephone, time-to-treatment was shorter and outcomes were the same. Besides, one day soon the emergency doctors and personnel in all these small hospitals would have to come to grips with tPA and learn to diagnose stroke. Why shouldn't they? What was the point of creating a system for consultation that would soon be obsolete?

"We know speed, accuracy, cost, and liability are factors," said Frey. "I posit the phone has the lead on all of these."

No clear winner emerged but there came a dramatic moment for telemedicine when, thrown up on the screen usually reserved for slides and charts, suddenly appeared a televised close-up of a distraught, confused elderly woman. Brett C. Meyer, the neurologist who directs the telemedicine program at the University of California, San Diego, had introduced himself to the patient by remote audio and video. He explained that he was 150 miles away but that did not matter.

"I'm zooming in on you right now so I can see you really, really well."

Probably not even a stroke, the emergency doctor had told him. He almost did not call—"But since I have you on the line…". As Meyer examined the woman visually and talked with her, the deficits were at first on the subtle side—but they were real and visible beyond the patient's evident disorientation. Meyer discerned a slight facial droop and weakness on her left side. Most interesting to him was the patient's problem with moving her eyes correctly. The woman, dressed in a drab hospital gown, actually grew worse during the evaluation. Her speech deteriorated even further, as did her strength. She was indeed having a stroke, and Meyer called for tPA.

Disconcerting as it was to bring a real-time acute stroke to a stroke meeting, still more remarkable was a jump-cut in the visual presentation that showed the same woman about 30 minutes after the drug was injected. Coherent speech had returned and she herself noted how her double vision was gone. At Meyer's instructions she looked to the right, to the left, and straight up.

"Perfect," said Meyer as the woman complied. "That's what we give the medicine for—to see people get better just like you. Thank you for getting better for me."

"Thank you," answered the woman.

If neither modality, telephone consult nor telemedicine, has a clear edge, each represents a valuable application when confidence of diagnosis is at issue. Each has potential problems in terms of liability and who gets paid for what. Both may lead to better care for acute stroke victims and at the same time— ideally, in fact—they will be limited to the medical margins when the day comes, if it comes, that tPA is in common and widespread use.

Unlike the vast majority of patients who want to put their stroke out of mind forever after, Julie Milanese tracked down the people who had helped her. She was grateful to her co-workers and her doctors. In particular, she sought out Ray Crawford, the paramedic who had brought her to the hospital. This proved awkward because Ray had violated the rules to send his ambulance miles out of the way to reach an ER where he knew she could receive tPA. Before Julie and her mother arrived to meet with him, he had to confess as much to his superior. He was reprimanded *pro forma* for not following protocol, but everybody knew it was ridiculous.

Julie not only thanked Ray but invited him to her wedding. Much as he found embarrassing any expression of gratitude, because paramedics are always forgotten once they deliver their patients to the emergency room, he was touched. His wife insisted they attend the reception at the lush Garden Court in San Francisco's venerable Palace Hotel.

"It was beautiful," he admitted. Seeing Julie was a huge satisfaction: "I could get lectured by the medical director of the state. But here's a woman who's standing in her wedding dress. And now she has no deficit."

It was, he said, unreal. But for all that it was unreal, for all the positive data and stars aligned, nothing so positive could be said about the numbers of patients treated.

Dawn Kleindorfer, a neurologist at the University of Cincinnati College of Medicine, faced not more than five or six reporters at Stroke 2009—not the dozens who would be on hand if this were the huge annual oncology or cardiovascular conference. She and colleagues had used a comprehensive database to track the number of times tPA was used to treat stroke patients between 2005 and 2007. A previous estimate had shown that a disappointing 1% of stroke victims received thrombolysis. Five years later, that figure had now doubled to a tad more than 2%. Meanwhile, 64% of all hospitals in the United States had not given tPA to *any* Medicare patients during the 2-year study period. These were mainly the ubiquitous small hospitals with fewer than 200 beds. The number of patients receiving tPA overall, said Kleindorfer, was flat from 2001 to 2004 prior to a bump upward in 2005, a year before improved, higher reimbursement Medicare rates went into effect.

"In the Cincinnati population, we get all the strokes in our region—a population of 1.3 million. And I know in that population, 8% are eligible. How many actually got treated? More like 4%." The disparity was hard to explain—maybe poor documentation by emergency doctors, perhaps system glitches; she did not know why. But whatever the precise reason, without a public health initiative, such low numbers are likely to persist.

The advent of tPA undoubtedly sped the development of primary stroke centers, comprehensive stroke centers, hub-and-spoke arrangements, and drip-and-ship capability. These were fine things. Eventually there was World Stroke Day and Stroke Awareness Day, and the month of May was proclaimed Stroke Awareness Month. But none of this translated into success in the central mission of raising consciousness about stroke among the population as a whole. Warning the public about the dangers of stroke while neglecting to point to the single treatment available, or to the time window in which to obtain it, did not prove to be a recipe for success—but for failure. Explanations might be various and valid: controversy over tPA, issues of infrastructure and administration, ingrained pessimism, and stroke's disorienting symptoms. But it was, and remains, a failure nonetheless and requires a fix.

Through the Looking Glass | 11

*E*ven as controversy among doctors diminished, the lack of widespread aware-ness of tPA or any willingness to think proactively about stroke have become the stuff of an upside-down, looking-glass world. More than 3,000 articles in medical journals alone have discussed thrombolysis and stroke, but tPA remains nearly invisible to people who most need to know about it. Exaggerated dangers of harm have overshadowed its demonstrable efficacy, which is all the more foolish because it is a one-time treatment—unlike drugs such as Vioxx or Fen-phen, which became dangerous when prescribed to large numbers of patients to be taken on a daily basis. Although tPA is unusually cost-effective, Medicare scarcely reimbursed hospitals for more than a decade and still leaves doctors under-compensated. In the United States neurologists were reluctant to protect the very organ they were trained to treat, while emergency doctors, popularly portrayed as aggressive cowboys in the ER, shrank from the idea of using a clot-dissolving drug to treat a brain attack.

By 2010, although many of these negatives were coming around at last, there remains a crucial paucity of interest on the part of those at risk. Besides cancer patients and their families, who frequently demand expensive treatments that do little good, pressure groups on behalf of patients with Alzheimer's dis-ease and amyotrophic lateral sclerosis (ALS, or Lou Gehrig's disease) generate considerable funding for a drug pipeline filled with hope but mostly empty of substance. Despite an aging population that portends a rising number of cases in decades to come, stroke remains an under-appreciated crippler and killer. Only a small minority know signs and symptoms and a scant few have heard of tPA. Fewer still know what they need to do to receive it.

To what extent public information campaigns that directly inform people about tPA would affect the number of patients seeking rapid treatment is unknown. In 2009 Dawn Kleindorfer and colleagues at the University of Cincinnati published results from a substantial series of telephone surveys. Asking open-ended questions about treatment for stroke, they found that just 62 of 2,156 respondents—under 3%—knew about tPA and were also aware they needed to seek treatment urgently. These results are all the more striking because the population surveyed in the greater Cincinnati/Northern Kentucky region is served by one of the most active stroke treatment groups in the nation. It is likely, writes Kleindorfer, that "the national and local campaigns that have been implemented have not been targeted appropriately to the audience nor tested for efficacy before implementation."

Most often, mention of tPA has been left out of public information campaigns. One can make a case for why: just 7 of 8 strokes are ischemic, so thrombolysis is not appropriate for all patients. Discussing tPA might compli-cate the message: a stroke is a stroke, first of all, and often lethal. Widespread awareness could mean more people demanding the drug even when it is not appropriate or if they are in a hospital not capable of giving it, or not willing to give it. Better that people just know the symptoms, call 911 immediately—and hope for the best. Today, such a rationale for silence around treatment has become questionable.

About 2007, mention of tPA, in fact, started to appear occasionally in some of the modest and usually not too effective public relations campaigns around stroke. Target audiences included African-Americans and women. The former, who are two to four times more likely to suffer stroke, were informed about tPA through a campaign that focused on educating schoolchildren, developed by the National Stroke Association (NSA). This would seem to represent a depar-ture for the NSA, whose major focus has been rehabilitation. Similarly, more women die of stroke than from cancer and AIDS combined, and the nonprofit Goddess Fund has begun dispensing information that is clear and concise and points explicitly to tPA.

Another sign linking tPA to stroke awareness has developed around the unsettling issue of finding an emergency venue where patients can receive treatment.

"Has your local hospital set up the appropriate steps for treating stroke as an emergency?" This question, from a campaign run by the American Stroke Association and known as Power to End Stroke, continues:

> One way to find out is by checking the Joint Commission's list of certified primary stroke centers. Local hospitals not currently on this list may still be prepared to treat stroke. Contact the emergency room administrator and ask if the hospital has acute stroke protocols that include guidelines for the use of tPA. Knowing which facilities are equipped to treat stroke can save valuable time.

Such sound advice, however, is more or less buried in an obscure website (http://www.powertoendstroke.org/stroke-recognize.html). Checking with local hospitals or contacting a professional organization requires effort and foresight likely to be made by only a self-selected few, unfortunately, but it is an excellent idea for individuals, families, and households. Every year several hundred thousand people are estimated to suffer a transient ischemic attack (TIA). That means, by definition, that they recover without apparent deficit, but they are at significantly heightened risk for a serious stroke in the future.

Stroke, to be sure, presents challenges in terms of reaching vulnerable populations, but small-bore campaigns must be complemented by much larger efforts to create awareness. There is yet to be mounted anywhere an effort comparable to, say, the high-profile campaigns to fight heart disease or breast cancer. There is nothing like Lance Armstrong's "Livestrong" wristbands for cancer research. For stroke, a comprehensive program would aim at creating mass and targeted campaigns both to inform people about stroke and to eliminate denial and resignation. It is reasonable to think that more than 200,000 victims each year in the United States alone could improve or recover completely. But tPA is actually used in just under 1/25th of all strokes.

Future scenarios present still more pressing reasons why universal awareness is so important. Although at present tPA remains the single FDA-approved drug, there will be new therapies for acute stroke. Clot-busting drugs themselves may be expected to improve. The tPA molecule can be modified in a variety of ways, provided with enhanced specificity for clots and perhaps less risk of bleeding. One such drug, tenecteplase, is already used to treat heart attack; however, recent federal budget restrictions interrupted trials planned for stroke. A novel thrombolytic drug derived from the venom of vampire bats failed in early trials but may still hold promise. Other drugs yet to be developed might be used alone or in combination with tPA to save brain tissue or lengthen the time-to-treatment window.

Devices to physically retrieve clots from blocked arteries without surgery are already in use, but their role is clouded. While some physicians use them, they have not been proven to be either effective or safe because the FDA, due to a longstanding quirk of the regulatory system, does not require it. Most patients considered for clot extraction will be outside the 3- to 4.5-hour window for treatment with tPA.

Similarly, angioplasty and stenting procedures have been designed to repair and strengthen cerebral arteries, and can be used either to prevent or treat a stroke. Angioplasty involves inserting a catheter equipped with a balloon that, when inflated, expands and re-opens the artery. Stenting refers to the placement within an artery of a reinforcing metal coil. Again, recent data showing safety and effectiveness for these procedures are tending positive but incomplete. Physicians already use them and so are reluctant to participate in randomized studies in which some patients would receive no treatment, even though the intervention might be more harmful than doing nothing. Another problem with all such procedures, at least for now and the foreseeable future, is that they are available in only a relatively small number of hospitals.

Imaging procedures have advanced in multiple ways since the 1980s, but new methods have not improved upon the use of CT for acute stroke. Physicians would like to believe that the newer imaging modalities, such as magnetic resonance imaging (MRI), can help determine which patients will benefit from thrombolysis, but so far they have not succeeded. In a significant number of cases, tPA will fail, but nobody has been able to predict beforehand who will not benefit from it.

Some novel drugs and device-driven therapies might also succeed in combination with tPA to save brain tissue or lengthen the time window to treatment. Laser treatment is one of these and is currently in trials; it is especially attractive for being essentially noninvasive. Cooling the brain—hypothermia—is similarly promising, though difficult and labor-intensive; several trials are under way. Cell therapy also holds promise, with treatments derived from either bone marrow or stem cells. But delivering new cells to the brain is problematic in itself, and such therapies may await a future generation.

All these treatments—and first of all tPA—contain a message about the nature of stroke that must be transmitted to the broadest possible public. Acute stroke itself is not likely to go away. Whatever advances there are in terms of prevention or treatment, stroke will remain an emergency. Quite like heart attack, it will be the way that many of us die. The challenge today is to eliminate from that ordinary fact the common perception of inevitability and feeling of resignation, to recognize instead the prospects for full recovery and the potential for avoiding disability—and a fate worse than death itself.

A fitting conclusion came with a telephone call Zivin received from Chicago in late 2009. Boris Vern, also a neurologist, was an old friend. He and Zivin had entered the same dual-degree medical scientist training program in the 1960s, and kept in touch ever after, meeting from time to time, hashing over ideas. A big soft-spoken man, Vern specialized in electrophysiology of the brain. When Zivin attended his daughter's wedding earlier in the year, Vern was talking about retiring from his full-time academic post at the University of Illinois at Chicago.

Now he phoned to say that just the other evening, shortly after returning home from a vacation in Europe—indeed, he had retired—while dozing in front of the television, he noticed his head seemed to be shaking. Then he found he could no longer move his left leg. Strange, that. Then his arm, he noticed, was clumsy. Wasn't that something? He tested his voice. He could talk but his speech was slurred.

At first, denial. It could be anything, he told himself, except a stroke. He was a neurologist, after all. His foot ought to behave itself or he was going to kick it. But after a moment it dawned on him: he was not being rational.

His son Peter and his wife Areta came to help. Areta, also a physician, was a specialist on a burn unit with a background in pathology and pediatric oncology. Her first thought when she saw her husband was: "He'll be back home in a wheelchair."

A team of emergency medics responded to 911 and transported Vern to Loyola University Medical Center. Of several local choices, it was the only one he trusted.

Vern did not much care for tPA. Much as he liked Zivin, he remained a skeptic. He knew the data but never fully believed them. But as the emergency medical team picked him up and brought him to the hospital—by this time, he estimated, if there was ever a call for tPA, this was it.

The doctors agreed. After an hour he still couldn't move the leg. His arm was weak and he felt like a drunken sailor. His symptoms were stable; he was not improving. A CT scan showed no bleed. He was eligible.

Vern's mind entered observational overdrive as he was treated. All right: he was not a big enthusiast. Indeed, he had reservations. But over the next 60 minutes, as the tPA dripped through the IV, Vern lay abed intently conscious. Nothing happened at first, and for some minutes. But gradually, the grip of paralysis disappeared. Then he was able to move his leg. As feeling was restored to it, he began to think about the drug less as tPA than as magic juice. He remembered Zivin.

"Jesus Christ, when I get out of here," he said to himself, "I'm going to call him." He even considered sending flowers, then nixed the idea: "That would be too much."

Within 6 hours strength and sensation had returned to his leg. Movement in his arm came back soon after; so did speech. Within 24 hours he was walking, talking, and normal. After leaving the hospital on his own a few days later, Vern did call Zivin, who was pleased to hear from him. As for the stroke, Zivin had heard it all before. Time and again.

Post-Script

The NINDS Stroke Study: A Personal Statement

My problems with the NINDS Stroke Study date to its very beginning. That I had trouble at all seems to me ironic because I have always considered myself a product of the National Institutes of Health (NIH), the parent organization of the National Institute of Neurological Disorders and Stroke (NINDS). Through NIH, my medical school and graduate school training were paid for as part of the Medical Scientists Training Program; in addition, I subsequently worked at NIH at the end of the Vietnam War, which fulfilled my military obligation. Those were two of the best years of my life, and my background there facilitated my early career. NIH has funded my research continuously for more than 30 years. I am truly grateful to the organization and view the NIH as a jewel in the federal government.

I was engaged in planning the NINDS trials for tPA for stroke from the start. In numerous discussions with John Marler, as mentioned in Chapter 4, I helped him, I believe, to design the official Request for Proposal (RFP). Together with his boss, Mike Walker, John hoped to jumpstart stroke therapy development by establishing a network of stroke centers around the country. Institutions would submit their credentials and, if selected, could apply to participate in studies as part of a Master Contract.

When the RFP was announced for the first pilot tPA trial, a phase I dose-finding effort, I had just moved to UCSD and was not yet well situated within the university. UCSD had no national reputation for stroke research, and it never occurred to me that we could join the Master Contract. About 2 weeks before the submission deadline, John called me to ask if La Jolla was somewhere near San Diego—unaware that it was at one time a separate town, but now is just a city neighborhood. As it turned out, John Alksne, then head of neurosurgery at UCSD with offices in La Jolla, had joined the Master Contract, so we were in fact eligible. Marler and I laughed about it at the time, but it meant a difficult couple of weeks. I tried as hard as I could to line everything up for a credible submission, but there was just not enough time. Reviewers at NINDS had no reason to think that we at UCSD were really any good at conducting clinical studies, and I personally had no reputation at that point as a clinical investigator. It was no surprise when our proposal was turned down.

Results of the phase I tPA stroke trial, as it turned out, seemed to me flawed. The specific reasons for my doubts are too technical to go into here, but the bottom line was that I viewed the selected dose of the drug as probably too low. Nevertheless, because I knew that tPA was so potent, using that dose for phase II testing (clinical trial protocol development) would be justified. When the opportunity arose to submit a proposal for that study, we at UCSD were ready. By then we had participated in other stroke trials and started to develop a national reputation. The phase I studies had included just three centers, but the planned phase II trial was to employ three times that number, so we had a much better chance of being accepted. Pat Lyden and I agreed it would help his career more than mine if he was to be the local principal investigator. I would be involved in the trial design and to some extent in patient recruitment, but he was going to do most of the work. When our proposal was accepted, we were very happy.

Problems for me, however, began with the first protocol development meeting. Many of us felt honored to be there, because we had confidence in the drug and thought this was going to be a historic trial (as it ultimately was), but I had little confidence in the results of the phase I trials and was not shy about letting my feelings be known. By then I had worked with the drug for 6 years and knew more about its effects in animal models and its pharmacology than anyone present. The Genentech representative, Steve Peroutka, understood how I felt and basically agreed with much of what I said, but he was only an observer. The various decisions about the protocol were made on the basis of a show of hands. Clinical investigators usually believe in what is called sweat equity: they are putting in the effort to conduct the clinical trials and therefore think their often shared opinions should predominate. But the best science is not done by a democratic process. I had one voice in a roomful of clinicians. In the hall during breaks, Steve and I would commiserate about some of the mistakes we thought were being made. Nevertheless, the final result was not terrible, and I very much wanted to participate in the trial.

All went reasonably well for the next 2 years. The trial proceeded toward a goal of treating 280 patients with placebo or tPA. In my estimation we would not need to treat that many patients because the efficacy of the drug was so great. I kept expecting the Data Safety and Monitoring Committee (DSMC) to terminate the trial almost any day. The DSMC is an independent group tasked with deciding if a trial should be stopped, whether because the drug is too dangerous or its efficacy is proven prior to completing patient recruitment.

Finally, after the full complement of 280 patients was recruited, I fully expected the results to be shared with the investigators and we would decide what to do next. What happened in fact was quite different. A meeting was called that brought together several of the local principal investigators, including Pat Lyden, the DSMC members, and representatives from NIH and Genentech. When Pat returned, he told me that a decision had been made: we were to recruit an additional 300 patients. Also, we should not question or even seriously discuss what was being done. We were expected simply to be good soldiers.

I was absolutely stunned. It took me a few days to think things through a little, and the more I thought about it, the more wrong the whole process seemed. This did not conform to the way that clinical trials were supposed to be conducted so far as I was concerned. What I viewed as a gag order was particularly offensive.

I did know a few facts. First, 280 patients (half treated with tPA and the other half with placebo) were apparently insufficient to convince the DSMC to terminate the trial as originally planned. But that made no sense to me: such committees were not supposed to decide protocol issues; they are simply independent groups charged with protecting patients from harm. Why would they unilaterally make decisions about continuing the trial? If NINDS as an organization was making an independent decision, they should have included the investigators in the process.

As it was, the trial had been set up in a unique way. Ordinarily, investigators propose clinical trials and a "Study Section"—a group of experts in the field working as advisors to NIH—conduct detailed reviews, offer recommendations, and usually make "suggestions" (really much stronger than that) about what should actually be done to improve the proposal. The investigators then use the review to make changes and resubmit it for further consideration. Although cumbersome and time-consuming, the process generally results in relatively good decisions. In this instance, with the study developed under the Master Contract, Mike Walker and John Marler were pretty much free to do as they wished without the constraints of expert opinion. I personally liked them but did not think that they should be making these types of decisions without outside assistance, at least from the investigators. Finally, I knew something else: we had been told that we needed to recruit another 300 patients.

With the information about the numbers of patients to be randomized, I was able to perform a statistical test known as a sensitivity analysis. There were two possibilities. One was that the trial had been successful and now we were being told to do a second trial before the results of the first were known. With tPA available in every emergency room in the country, I thought that withholding information that it worked for stroke was unacceptable. At the time, I actually did not take that possibility seriously because I did not think the people in charge would do such a thing. However, the alternate possibility, as indicated by my statistical analysis, showed that if 600 patients were required to prove tPA was effective, the drug would not be used because neurologists would view its efficacy as too weak to justify the perceived risk. Since I did not trust either the results of the phase I study or the process by which the phase II protocol had been developed, I thought the study should be redesigned. A second trial without exposing results of the first was unacceptable as far as I was concerned; so too was a continuation that would only demonstrate weak efficacy. But I was not sure what action to take.

It was an especially uncomfortable time for me. My research depended on my receiving NINDS grant support, and Mike Walker and John Marler were the people who were my oversight at NIH. Making enemies of them would be distinctly unhelpful to my future in research. However, I really did not think I had a choice. Someday people would look back on how we conducted the trials and potentially question what we did. I hated the idea of challenging the "gag order" but knew I had to do it.

These events occurred in early 1993, not long before the yearly International Stroke Conference sponsored by the American Heart Association. It is the largest stroke meeting held in the United States, and I knew all the players would be there. In particular, Mike Walker would attend, and I wanted to talk with him face to face. I brought my sensitivity analysis and, very nervously when I saw him at the beginning of the meeting, I asked him to look it over, along with a one-page discussion about my concerns. He took the documents and we parted. I did not talk to him again until 2 days later, when he came up to me, handed me the papers, and told me to get rid of them. There was little other discussion that I can remember. The meeting ended and I went home.

The next day, I received a call from John Marler. He told me that he and Mike had decided that I had a conflict of interest. They knew I had been working with Genentech on my animal studies and provided the company with additional advice about the clinical development strategy for tPA for stroke. I did not own any Genentech stock and my consulting arrangement paid me very little. However, Mike and John now decided that I was a liability to the trial because of my relationship to the company. It seemed obvious that my challenge was being answered with a sudden demand that I quit the trial. Furthermore, I feared that they could try to retaliate by eliminating my research funding. I did as they asked and promptly resigned from the trial. For weeks thereafter I felt awful. However, I did not get rid of the papers I had given to Mike—I had them notarized.

I certainly had the option of stirring up trouble by complaining to the other investigators or, possibly, going to the newspapers to try to air my concerns. Ultimately I decided that this path would hurt development of the drug, and that was the last thing I wanted. Also, I could not be sure which of my interpretations of the trial was correct. So I decided to do nothing. Mike and John took no additional punitive action. John and I had been friends before all of this happened, but our relationship afterwards was never the same. I did not blame him for forcing me to resign: he and Mike were trying to conduct the trial with as little internal conflict as possible, making me the nail sticking up that had to be hammered flat.

For almost exactly 2 years the trial proceeded as before. During that period, among other things, I helped form CerebroVascular Advances (CVA), a contract research company that helped conduct clinical studies. CVA specialized in acute stroke trials, originally exclusively with drugs. A drug maker or device manufacturer would hire CVA and we would provide expertise to help them develop the protocol, collect data accurately, and analyze the results. When the trial was over, the company could terminate its relationship with CVA and, as a result, did not need to fire any of its own employees. Physician investigators enjoyed working with us because, being so specialized, we thoroughly understood the problems they encountered and, among other services, provided knowledgeable and prompt answers to their questions. When trying to recruit stroke patients into trials with very strict time-to-treatment requirements, for example, to be able to contact a source of accurate information about study protocols at any hour of the day or night has genuine value.

During that 2-year period, I kept track of the NINDS trial by periodically talking with our nurses, who were always kept up to date about how many patients had been recruited. I knew very little more. However, in January 1995, the second phase of the NINDS tPA study ended. At that point I was surprised that no announcement was made, at least concerning the first half of the trial. I just did not know what to think.

Nothing more happened until the end of summer 1995 when, shortly after the Airlie meeting described in Chapter 4, I received a call from a clinical scientist with Genentech. He wanted to talk confidentially and told me, somewhat indirectly, that the trial had been successful and Genentech now wanted help in completing its own trial. The NINDS tPA trial had recruited patients only if they could be treated within 3 hours after stroke onset. Genentech wanted to see if it was possible to extend the window to 5 hours, but their trial was going poorly. He wanted CVA to take over its operation, and we were happy to comply. Now I was aware of the outcome of the NINDS tPA trial but did not know the magnitude of the success.

In late fall I received a request from John Marler for an immediate meeting in Bethesda, Maryland. John was always secretive, so such a call from him was not particularly surprising, but I had no idea what it was about. We met on a weekend morning and he took me to a small cafeteria restaurant for brunch. After we got our food and sat down, he handed me a preprint of the article describing the NINDS trials, soon to be published in the *New England Journal of Medicine* and later to become a classic in the field of stroke therapy. I was happy to see both how big the effect size of tPA was and how safe it was, and I congratulated him and the investigators. However, I quickly looked for the information that told whether the first part of the trial—at the termination of which I had been forced to resign—had been as successful as the second part. When I saw that there was essentially no difference between the two cohorts of patients, I became nauseated. All I could think of was the stroke victims who had been effectively denied treatment for some 2 years while the second part of the trial, which I opposed, had been conducted. I did not finish eating but said nothing about how I was feeling at that point.

Several weeks later, after the article was published, I saw John again at the International Stroke Meeting. By this time I had regained my composure and simply asked him about some of the decisions that had been made at the time I thought the trial should have ended. He said they had decided that they wanted conclusive proof the drug worked and that the FDA had insisted on a second placebo-controlled trial. He added that if they had released the information after the first 280 patients, the investigators may well have refused to conduct a second trial because they would have known there was such strong proof that the drug actually worked. As a member of the FDA panel that reviewed neurological drugs, I knew that there existed no requirement for a second trial. The FDA sometimes requested a second trial but did not invariably demand one.

That the agency always did demand one was a common belief, at the time and even now, but it was incorrect.

In summary, the results of the first trial should have been released 2 years before they were. Alternatively, even if one accepts the argument that a second trial was needed, I can see no excuse for sitting on the data from the first trial after recruitment of patients for the second trial ended. The final patient visits occurred in January 1995, almost a year before the article in the *New England Journal of Medicine* was published.

In general, I believe Mike Walker and John Marler exercised more influence over the conduct of the trial than they would later claim. I also take issue with the belief, which some investigators shared, that results of the study should not have been released prior to publication. Concern that doctors in clinical practice would use tPA off-label without first informing themselves of any risks was, in my view, quite unfounded.

The FDA panel of outside advisors met in the early summer of 1996 when the results of the NINDS study, together with the original source documents, were presented with a request to make acute ischemic stroke an indication for treatment with tPA. The FDA is not required to accept the advice of this panel, and has not done so concerning some politically sensitive drugs (especially those for birth control), but disagreement is rare. Since I was a member of the panel, I declared that here I really did have a conflict of interest and recused myself. But because other drugs were being reviewed by my panel at that same meeting, the FDA invited me to attend; I simply did not participate in the discussions about tPA. In my place for that particular part of the meeting sat John Hallenback, a leading stroke investigator working at NIH and a good friend. I was required to sit in the FDA section of the audience and was specifically prohibited from any interaction with Genentech. I felt gagged and manacled because I so badly wanted to answer some of the questions under discussion.

During that meeting I was nervous. All through its development tPA had been exceptionally controversial, and some of the country's most prominent neurologists first wanted additional studies. Nevertheless, FDA approval was unanimous. The vote was conducted by having the panel members raise their hands to affirm the recommendation. I remember it as one of the proudest moments of my professional life.

The day before the meeting I helped the people from Genentech prepare their oral presentations. When the outcome was successful, they took us out for a celebration at the Hay-Adams Hotel, near Lafayette Park across from the White House. Dinner was very good, but I was aware that a similar if less elegant affair was taking place among the trial investigators, and in many ways I would rather have been with them.

After approval, issues I had feared concerning acceptance indeed came to pass. I believe that if the trial had been ended after the first cohort of 280 patients, many of these problems could have been minimized or avoided, and any controversy might have been short-lived. To view the NINDS tPA study as a single trial was a major misperception on the part of critics, and their argument that the trials needed to be replicated was fallacious. But in the case of a drug as controversial as tPA, for many, perception would become reality. That the NINDS tPA study was in fact two separate trials was rendered ambiguous by the way the results were presented in a single article in the *New England Journal of Medicine*. Had the results of the first part of the trial been revealed as soon as it was over, as I believe they should have been, a second placebo-controlled trial could have been conducted. A positive outcome might have ensured more rapid acceptance. At the time, we predicted to Genentech that the neurology community would require several years to make the radical changes required to treat strokes as emergencies.

In the final analysis, however, there were no villains in this story. All involved thought they were doing what was best, but the result, in my opinion, was that over the years an untold number of stroke victims, perhaps millions, were denied an opportunity to receive a therapy that may have substantially benefited them. In 1994, tPA was available in virtually every emergency venue in the United States and was a welcome treatment for heart attack. Although NINDS study administrators could not have foretold the future of tPA, had they released the results of the first trial when they were available, everyone would have been better served and controversy, not the drug itself, might well have been marginalized.

In the end, I am pleased that tPA acute stroke therapy has at last moved toward consensus among responsible physicians. This book represents a major effort on my part to rectify the longstanding resistance to its use and to bring about widespread awareness that patients are routinely not being offered what is still the only effective treatment for acute stroke. A variety of efforts are currently bringing the treatment into the mainstream, giving it the standard-of-care status that it has deserved all along. If this book contributes to that end, if it reaches patients and physicians and helps to effect systemic change, I will feel it has really accomplished my main goal.

J.A.Z.
November 20, 2009

Interviews

All interviews were conducted by JGS, by telephone unless indicated (*) as face-to-face.

Harold P. Adams Jr., MD
Professor and Director, Division of Cerebrovascular Disorders, University of Iowa
  Stroke Center

Fedor Bachman, MD
Emeritus Professor, Department of Medicine, University of Lausanne

William George Barsan, MD
Professor and Chair, Department of Emergency Medicine, University of Michigan

William F. Bennett, PhD
Senior Director of Regulatory Science and Policy Assessment, Genentech

Joseph P. Broderick, MD
Professor and Chairman, Director, Greater Cincinnati/Northern Kentucky Stroke
  Team; Department of Neurology, College of Medicine, University of Cincinnati

Thomas G. Brott, MD
Department of Neurology, Mayo Clinic College of Medicine, Jacksonvile, Florida

Alastair Buchan, MD
Head of the Medical Sciences Division, University of Oxford

Louis R. Caplan, MD
Professor of Neurology at Harvard Medical School and Chief of the Stroke Service at
    the Beth Israel Deaconess Medical Center

Yu-Feng Yvonne Chan, MD
Associate Professor of Emergency Medicine, Mount Sinai School of Medicine,
    New York

Désiré Collen, MD, PhD
Director of the Molecular Cardiovascular Medicine Group (comprising the Center for
    Molecular and Vascular Biology of the K.U. Leuven, and the Center for Transgene
    Technology and Gene Therapy of the Flanders Interuniversity Institute for
    Biotechnology) in Leuven, Belgium

David Drachman, MD
Professor and Chairman Emeritus, Department of Neurology, University of
    Massachusetts Medical Center

J. Donald Easton, MD
Professor and Chairman, Department of Clinical Neurosciences, Brown
    Medical School

Jonathan A. Edlow, MD
Associate Professor of Medicine; Vice Chair, Department of Emergency Medicine,
    Beth Israel Deaconess Medical Center

Marc Fisher, MD
Professor of Neurology and Radiology, and Vice Chairman, Department of Neurology,
    University of Massachusetts Medical School

Elliott Grossbard, MD
Executive Vice President and Chief Medical Officer, Rigel Pharmaceuticals; formerly
    Director, Clinical Research, Genentech

James C. Grotta, MD
Professor and Chairman, Department of Neurology, University of Texas Medical
    School at Houston, and Director, Stroke Program, Memorial Hermann-Texas
    Medical Center

Vladimir Hachinski, MD, FRCP(C), DSc
Professor of Neurology, University of Western Ontario

Werner Hacke, MD, PhD
Professor and Chairman, Department of Neurology, University
    of Heidelberg

Jerome R. Hoffman, MD
Professor of Clinical and Emergency Medicine at the David Geffen School of Medicine,
    University of California, Los Angeles

Steven H. Horowitz, MD
Neurologist, Yarmouth, ME; formerly Department of Neurology, Long Island Jewish
    Medical Center

Andy S. Jagoda, MD
Professor and Chair, Department of Emergency Medicine, Mount Sinai School of
    Medicine, New York

Markku Kaste, MD
Professor Emeritus, Department of Neurology, Helsinki University Central Hospital,
    University of Helsinki

Kennedy Lees, MD, FRCP*
Professor of Cerebrovascular Medicine, University of Glasgow; Director, Acute Stroke
    Unit, Western Infirmary

Jeanne Lenzer
Freelance journalist

Steven R. Levine, MD*
Professor and Vice Chair of Neurology, State University of New York Health Science
    Center; formerly Clinical Associate Professor of Neurology, Henry Ford Health
    Sciences Center

Didier Leys
Professor of Neurology and Head of the Department of Neurology, Lille University
    Hospital, chairman of the French Stroke Society (1998–2000), and current
    President of the European Stroke Organisation

James Li, MD
Director, Remote Medical Service Field Course and Assistant Professor of Emergency
    Medicine, Harvard School of Medicine

Eugene D. Locken, DO, JD
Physician and attorney, Santa Barbara, California

Patrick D. Lyden, MD*
Chair, Department of Neurology, Cedars-Sinai Medical Center; formerly Professor of
    Clinical Neurology and served as the Clinical Chief of Neurology and Director of
    the Stroke Center, University of California, San Diego Medical Center

John E. Markis, MD
Assistant Clinical Professor of Medicine, Harvard Medical School

John R. Marler, MD*
Neurologist, Bethesda, MD; Medical Officer, FDA; formerly Associate Director
    for Clinical Trials, National Institute of Neurological Disorders and Stroke

Brett C. Meyer, MD
Associate Professor of Clinical Neurosciences, University of California,
    San Diego Medical Center and Medical Director for the Department
    of Telemedicine

Diane Pennica, PhD
Senior Scientist, Genentech

Stephen J. Peroutka
Neurologist; formerly Director of Clinical Research, Department of
    Neuroscience, Genentech

Jean Range
Executive Director, Disease-Specific Care Certification, Joint Commission

Daniel B. Rifkin, PhD
Charles Aden Poindexter Professor of Medicine, New York University

Jack E. Riggs, MD
Vice Chair, Department of Neurology, West Virginia University

Ralph Sacco, MD
Miller School of Medicine, University of Miami; President, American
    Heart Association

Peter Sandercock, MD, FRCP*
Department of Clinical Neurosciences, Western General Hospital, Edinburgh

Philip A. Scott, MD
Associate Professor, Department of Emergency Medicine, University of Michigan

Jeffrey Saver, MD*
Professor of Neurology, UCLA School of Medicine; Director, UCLA Stroke Center

Vineeta Singh, MD
Assistant Professor of Clinical Neurology, University of San Francisco Medical Center

Joan A. Stashak, MS

Barbara C. Tilley, PhD
Professor and Director, Division of Biostatistics, School of Public Health, University of
    Texas Health Science Center, Houston; formerly Principal Investigator,
    Coordinating Center, NINDS Stroke Trial, Henry Ford Health Sciences Center

Eric Topol, MD
Professor of Translational Genomics, Department of Molecular and Experimental
    Medicine, Scripps Research Institute

Boris A. Vern, MD
Associate Professor and Director, Section of Narcolepsy and Sleep Disorders in the
    Department of Neurology and Rehabilitation, University of Illinois at Chicago

Michael D. Walker
Formerly Director, Division of Stroke, Trauma, and Neurodegenerative Disorders,
    NINDS

Charles Warlow, MD, FRCP
Professor of Medical Neurology, Department of Clinical Neurosciences, Western
    General Hospital, Edinburgh

K. M. A. Welch, MD, FRCP
President and CEO, Rosalind Franklin University of Medicine and Science;
    formerly Head, Coordinating Center, NINDS Stroke Trial, Henry Ford
    Health Science Center

Takenori Yamaguchi, MD
National Cardiovascular Center, Suita, Osaka, Japan

Notes

To the Reader

xi. "five million people..." Statistics from the World Health Organization. See http://www.strokecenter.org/patients/stats.htm

xii. Mark J. Alberts, quoted in *The New York Times* (May 28, 2007)

Chapter 1 Code Stroke on Market Street

The narrative in this chapter is based on interviews with Julie Milanese Jensen, Ray Crawford, Doug Jensen, Steve Kondonijakos, Ericka Milanese, Rick Milanese, and Vineeta Singh, MD.

5. "It was sort of..." Drachman interview 3/21/2007

5. President Woodrow Wilson... Fields and Lemak (1989), 192

5. "came out of the..." Henig (1997), 134

7. One study from Israel... Rozenthul-Sorokin et al. (1996)

8. Only in 1905... Owen (2001), Chapter 6

Chapter 2 Clot-buster: The Natural History

13. Alfons Billiau... The story of the first clinical use of tPA (at the time called HEPA) is assembled from personal accounts found in H. R. Lingen et al., the privately published *Désiré Collen: An Anthology of Scientific Collaborations* (2008). See also Collen and Lingen (2004).

13. "Ever heard of HEPA?..." Ibid. 124. Language as quoted confirmed by W. Weimar, personal communication (WW/JGS) (6/24/2009)

14. "The clot completely dissolved..." Ibid. 124

14. "The case was reminiscent..." Ibid. 19

14. "gift from nature..." Le Fanu (2002), 14

14. Alexander Fleming... Fleming's perspicacity as a scientist has long been a source of some dispute among both scientists and historians of medicine. See Bud (2007) for an excellent discussion of the discovery of penicillin in relation to a scientific collaboration, industry, and medicine.

15. "decisively influenced..." Collen (1996), 861

15. "long anticipated therapeutic..." Porter (1997), 458

15. "chambers of horror..." Fletcher, quoted in Le Fanu (2002), 7

15. "end of a mandate..." Starr (1982), Chapter 4

16. The bare discovery... Astrup and Permin (1947)

16. Long on promise... See Mueller and Scheidt (1994); Sikri and Bardia (2007).

17. "In 1949..." Sherry (1989), 1085

17. "was based on...." Ibid. 1086-7

17. For stroke, the promise... Meyer, Barnhart, and Johnson (1965)

18. "It must be concluded...." Genton et al. (1977), 173

18. In the 1840s... Virchow (1997); see also Schiller (1970)

18. "thrombi may be..." Roberts (1972), 222

18. This interpretation became... Maroo and Topol (2004); Weisse (2006)

18. In 1980 Marcus DeWood... Maroo and Topol (2004); see also Sikri and Bardia (2007)

19. "Intractable all these..." The narrative of the extraction, purification, and subsequent genetic sequencing of tPA is based on interviews with Désiré Collen, Daniel Rifkin, and Diane Pennica, with further confirmation provided by Fedor Bachman. See also Collen and Lingen (2004) and Lingen et al. (2008).

21. Producing pure tPA... Rijken and Collen (1981); Rijken, Hoylaerts, and Collen (1982)

21. Collen sketched a larger... Collen (1996)

22. "important consequences..." Ibid.

22. In 1979, when Désiré Collen... See the classic account of Genentech's early years in Hall (1987).

23. Persuaded by the head… Bera (2009), 760. The reference is to Niels Reimers, founder of Stanford University's technology commercialization program.

23. Genentech's actual decision… See Heyneker and Hughes (2002).

23. "sounds even more interesting…" Quoted in Kleid and Hughes (2002)

24. The science at Genentech… Bazell (1998), 45: "As Genentech matured from its arrogant youth into the adult real world of drug development, it coped by splitting its corporate personality in half. The science remained excellent."

24. Collen was skeptical… See Pennica's account in Lingen et al. (2008), 82.

24. Yet Pennica was… Ibid.

24. she was young and attractive…. On Pennica's looks and demeanor, see Kleid and Hughes (2002).

24. "I didn't tell him…" Pennica in Lingen et al. (2008)

24. She would present… Pennica et al. (1983)

Chapter 3   Dead or Alive

27. "I trained with…" JAZ/JGS interview 3/7/2007

27. "He wanted to do a clot…." Grossbard interview 5/1/2007

28. "Biotechnology is more…." Montgomery (1983), 1

28. "There are times…" Ibid. 27

28. "the first practical way…" Ibid. 47

29. "Those were data…." JAZ/JGS interview 11/25/08

29. "Physically, it was…" Ehrenhalt (1996), 39

30. "He probably set up…" Drachman interview 3/21/2007

31. In fact, several recent advances… See, e.g., Plum (1983).

31. "No specific drug…" Hachinski and Norris (1985), 230

31. "[F]rom the standpoint…" Baker (1962), 830

32. "popgun pharmacy…." Osler (1908), 82

32. "Diane Pennica…." Pennica interview 2/4/2009

32. "appropriate types of stroke…" Correspondence, Zivin to Grossbard, 1/27/1984

32. "Although interesting…" Correspondence, Marafino to Zivin, 2/13/1984

33. Although Zivin was not… Grossbard interview 5/1/2007

33. "I thought that at…." Ibid.

33. Absence of a treatment… See, e.g., Raichle (1982).

33. "The well-contained fire…" Hass (1983); see Hachinski and Norris (1985), 51

33. Recent research challenged… Plum (1983); Zivin (1998)

34. A time window… Zivin (1982)

34. "pharmacologic strategies..." Ibid. 412

34. "I was stuck..." JAZ/JGS interview 1/30/2007

34. Indeed, the animal models... See, e.g., Stefanovich (1982).

35. *Quantal dose-response analysis...* See Zivin and Waud (1992).

35. "one asks detailed..." Virchow (1958), 37

35. "If you made something..." JAZ/JGS interview 2/19/2009

36. "Statistics for Disinterested..." Zivin (1976)

36. one of which... Zivin and Waud (1982)

37. "In baseball, you..." JAZ/JGS interview 2/20/2009

38. "If this goes..." JAZ/JGS interview 3//7/2007

38. "And I wait..." Quoted in Simmons (2002), 20

38. "high context" activity... E. Hall (1976), 91ff. Hall, a cultural anthropologist, distinguishes between "low context" messages (an airline schedule, for example) and "high context" communication in which "most of the information is either in the physical context or internalized in the person...".

38. "When I saw..." Joan Stashak interview 1/20/2009

39. Impressive numbers stood out.... Zivin (1985)

39. "Those guys..." JAZ/JGS interview 1/9/2009

40. "the statistical literature..." Zivin and Waud (1982), 1407

40. "Although it may sound..." See, e.g., Matthews and McPherson (1987); West and Ficalora (2007).

40. Other research tended... Del Zoppo et al. (1986); Del Zoppo (1988)

Chapter 4 Brain-O

41. "Tom Brott came armed..." Barbara Tilley interview 8/29/2007

41. "Nevertheless, the place struck..." Patrick Lyden interview 4/7/2007

41. He had chosen Airlie... John Marler interview 2/20/2009

42. "We all assembled..." Lyden interview 4/7/2007

42. "Well, we did it..." Ibid.

42. "Open the Champagne..." Ibid.

43. "It was a remarkable..." K. Michael Welch interview 4/10/2009

43. "In cancer..." Lyden interview 2/19/2009

44. "consistent and persuasive..." Minutes of the NINDS Monitoring Committee Meeting (December 4, 1992)

44. In 1978...one clinical trial... Rowland (2003), 113

44. "None of the basic..." Walker interview 10/27/2008

45. Zivin met Marler... Marler interview 2/20/2009

45. What crystallized for Marler… Jones et al. (1981)

45. Zivin, who learned of this work… Zivin (1998)

46. "needed a friend…" Marler interview 11/10/2008

46. "You can't imagine…" Ibid.

46. "We thought we would…" Brott interview 4/16/2007

46. He knew he had convinced… JAZ/JGS interview 6/17/2009; correspondence: William F. Bennett to Jordan Gutterman, Lasker Foundation, January 26, 1996

47. "The reason we're giving…" Marler interview 2/20/2009

47. "We would get a page…" Brott interview 4/16/2007

48. "Clearly, additional larger…" Haley et al. (1993)

48. It "looked interesting and…" Walker interview 10/27/2008

49. To decide on participating… Marler interview 2/20/2009

50. "Every emergency department…" Tilley interview 8/29/2007; see also Tilley et al. (1997)

50. "We drew up Deming…" Welch interview 4/10/2009

50. "There was a real…" Steven H. Horowitz interview 3/25/2009

50. "I'd probably be playing…" Steven R. Levine interview 8/1/2007

50. "Whether because of Justin's…" Lyden interview 2/18/2009

51. "They literally laughed…" Ibid.

51. "I had my car equipped…" Ibid.

51. "We were seeing…" Lyden interview 2/19/2009

52. "I had never done…" Lyden interview 6/10/2009

53. "It was with a sinking…" Welch interview 4/10/2009

53. "They at the time had…" Walker interview 10/27/2008

54. By 1991 several powerful… See Robbins-Roth (2000)

54. "whenever possible to measure…" Quoted in Miller (1997) 93

54. Walker and other members… J. Donald Easton interview 4/10/2009

54. "We had a situation…" Lyden interview 2/18/2009

54. "Did that mean we…" Ibid.

54. "this dive, almost a Motel 6…" Lyden interview 2/18/2009

55. "extraordinary complexity and sensitivity…" Minutes of the NINDS Monitoring Committee Meeting (December 4, 1992)

55. "You had to pick…" Walker interview 10/27/2008

55. "were making it progressively…" Minutes December 4, 1992

55. "kind of against all…" Marler interview 2/20/2009

55. "came to us with…" Ibid.

55. "We're all committed to…" Lyden interview 2/18/2009

56. "interests, concerns, worries…" Minutes of the NINDS Monitoring Committee Meeting (December 4, 1992)

56. "quite mysterious..." Lyden interview 2/18/2009

56. "that their concerns about safety..." Minutes December 4, 1992

57. "We ran what were...." Walker interview 10/27/2008

57. "The [DSMC] did an incredibly..." Ibid.

58. "How Dachman came to......" Dr. Dachman did not respond to telephone requests or a request by mail to discuss her work on the NINDS Stroke Study.

58. "absolute complete joy..." Welch interview 4/10/2009

59. "And you just know..." Lyden interview 2/19/2009

59. "Tilley also noted..." Tilley interview 8/29/2007

Chapter 5 The Brain Doctors Cometh—Slowly

63. "If I'm driving through..." Don Easton interview 4/10/2009

63. "We thought this would..." Levine interview 8/1/2007

64. a few months after... NINDS r-tPA Stroke Study Group (1995)

64. a thrombolysis meeting took place... Fourth International Symposium on Thrombolytic Therapy for Acute Ischemic Stroke, 30 May–1 June, 1996, Copenhagen, Denmark. See *Cerebrovascular Diseases* 1996;6:175-94.

65. "under what current circumstances..." Anthony J. Furlan (1997), 215

65. a roundtable discussion of... See *Cerebrovascular Diseases*, Ibid., p. 78. Interviews: JAZ/JGS 5/29/2009, Lyden 6/10/2009.

65. "If any of you have a stroke..." JAZ/JGS interview, Ibid.

66. "Thrombolysis—Not a Panacea..." Caplan et al. (1997) The "Clinical Debate" entitled "Should Thrrombolytic Therapy Be the First-Line Treatment for Acute Ischemic Stroke" includes the article by Caplan et al and the response by Grotta. http://content.nejm.org/cgi/content/full/337/18/1309

66. "We think," they wrote..." Ibid.

66. "Although time is important,..." Ibid.

66. Responding, Jim Grotta... Grotta (1997)

67. "Nor should such academic concerns..." Ibid.

67. "I didn't really think debate..." Grotta interview 2/18/2009

67. "We probably use more tPA..." Ibid.

67. "We promised that if you came..." Lyden interview 2/19/2009

68. Studies consistently showed... See, e.g., Lattimore (2003); Edwards (2007).

68. In separate 1997 articles... Tilley (1997) and Broderick (1997)

68. they were "salivating...."Andrew Pollack (1988)

68. " 'Neurologists,' said Pat Lyden,..." Lyden interview 2/19/2009

68. "So all these guys..." Horowitz interview 3/25/2009

69. "We think of ourselves..." Ibid.

69. "The clinical responsibility for diagnosis..." Goldstein (2008), 47

69. "Neurologists, Get Off Your Hands!" Horowitz (1988)

69. "to convey my impressions..." Ibid. 155

69. "My personal belief is..." Ibid. 157

70. "Emergency medicine physicians and..." Ibid. 156

70. "I don't know how many..." Grotta interview 2/18/2009

70. "Tissue-Type Plasminogen Activator..." Jack E. Riggs (1997)

70. "a pedantic discussion of..." Horowitz, Ibid. 156

70. "risk of early iatrogenic..." Riggs, Ibid. 103

71. Thrombolysis for whatever... Thrombolytic therapy in thrombosis: a National Institutes of Health consensus development conference. *Annals of Internal Medicine* July 1980;93(1):141-4. Also published in other venues.

72. "Our current understanding..." Lyden and Zivin (1993), 13

72. He went on.... Zivin (1990)

72. Genentech scientists had taken... Correspondence: G. Roger Thomas to Jordan Gutterman, Albert and Mary Lasker Foundation, 1/24/1996

72. In 1951 C. Miller Fisher and Raymond D. Adams... Lyden and Zivin (1993)

73. From 1987 to 1991 Zivin and Pat Lyden... Ibid. 4-6

73. Zivin confirmed earlier research... Ibid. 7

73. "transformation is of little concern..." Ibid. 13

74. "We were very, very, very..." Welch interview 4/10/2009

74. "the 6 percent in whom..." Hadler (2008), 30

74. "No issue has caused greater..." Donnan and Davis (2003), 372

74. They had concluded.... Ibid. with reference to Donnan and Davis (2001)

74. "unusually positive and in general..." Lindley (2001), 2708

74. "have been digested, criticized..." Lyden (2001), 2710

75. the European Cooperative Acute Stroke Study (ECASS)... Hacke et al. (1995)

75. "The Alteplase Thrombolysis for Acute Noninterventional Therapy in Ischemic Stroke (ATLANTIS)..." Clark et al. (1999)

75. trials were pooled and showed... Hacke et al. (2004)

75. In 1999 the NINDS Stroke Study... Kwiatkowski et al. (1999)

75. a so-called phase IV trial... Albers et al. (2000)

75. One study, out of the Cleveland... Katzan (2000)

75. 4 years later published... Katzan (2003)

76. "We use tPA all the time...." Riggs interview 5/13/2009

76. "I'm still not overly impressed with its utility...." Ibid.

76. "Approval of tPA..." Caplan (2009), 162

76. the clock "doesn't make any sense to me..." Louis R. Caplan interview 3/16/2009

76. "Steadily accumulating data..." J. P. Mohr (2000), 1189

76. "Looking back..." Furlan (2000), 1451

76. "It might be easier..." Welch interview 4/10/2009

Chapter 6 What Emergency?

79. "some guy from California..." Horowitz interview 3/25/2009

79. "relies little on fact..." Marler interview 2/20/2009

80. "They were all over it..." Barsan interview 8/12/2009

80. "A lot of ER docs thought..." Ibid.

80. "It was bred by new..." Zink (2005), 11

81. He belonged to its first generation... Scheck (2003), 4. For the record, Jerome Hoffman was interviewed on two occasions for this book. He requested that we not use material from those interviews in this book and we have respected his wishes.

81. "a force in emergency medicine..." Ibid.

81. "played a big role in..." Zink (2005), 266

81. "odd man out..." Sheck, Ibid.

81. "[T]he importance of the syndrome..." McElroy and Hoffman (1981)

82. documentary entitled *Money Talks*... http://www.moneytalksthemovie.com/

82. "rarely save (really save)..." Hoffman's preface to Brown (1997), xviii

82. "'Tell me realistically,' he asked..." Interviews: Marler 11/10/08; Barsan 8/12/2009. The conversation as reconstructed was recollected by Barsan, confirmed by Marler.

82. he injected the first patient... Barson interview 8/12/2009

82. "'It used to be,' Barsan recalls..." Ibid.

83. "There is no diagnostic dilemma..." Philip A. Scott interview 4/2/2009

83. "Basically we were the people..." Barsan interview 8/12/2009

84. "could only help, at most,..." Hoffman (2000), 149

84. "the benefit [in the NINDS Study]..." Hoffman (2003), 333

84. "An even greater concern..." Hoffman (2000), 149-50

85. "And just what is the emperor..." Ibid.

85. It was a well-known story... Shortly before his death in 1993, Sol Sherry in his autobiography (1992) complained bitterly about the development of tPA for heart attack. Linda Marsa (1997) made the story one of several recounted in a muckraking effort, *Prescription for Profits* (1997). Aspects of the controversy were discussed in the literature from the late 1980s and also reported in the popular press. But also see also Sobel (1997), *Tissue Plasminogen Activator In Thrombolytic Therapy*, edited by cardiologist Burton Sobel, Désiré Collen, and Elliott Grossbard. Oral histories of the development of tPA at

Genentech for heart attack and stroke are also available at the Program in the History of the Biological Sciences and Biotechnology, available through the Bancroft Library of the University of California, Berkeley: http://bancroft.berkeley.edu/ROHO/projects/biosci/oh_list.html

85. "[W]e should all ask why…" Hoffman (2000), 150

85. "[I]n the absence of studies…" Hoffman (2003), 333

85. three randomized stroke trials… These were the Australian Streptokinase Trial (ASK), the Multicentre Acute Stroke Trial–Italy (MAST-ITALY), and the Multicentre Acute Stroke Trial–Europe (MAST-E).

86. Streptokinase provokes low blood… See, e.g., Cornu (2000).

86. "Further trials with [streptokinase]…" Ibid. 1560

86. leaders had quashed Genentech's hopes… Brott interview 4/16/2007

87. "Alteplase for Stroke…" Lenzer (2002)

87. "treatment recommendation that could…" Ibid. 723

87. had gleefully reported the essentials… In their column of November 10, 2000, according to Mokhiber (e-mail to JGS 2/18/2010), on the Focus on the Corporation Web site. See http://www.jacksonprogressive.com/issues/mokhiberweissman/genetech11100.html

87. "deprived the scientific community…" Lenzer (2002), 725

88. "with only 0.4% of patients…" Ibid. 723

88. "bloated claims…" Ibid.

88. "The term…" Ibid. 724

88. "chance alone could explain…" Ibid. 723

88. "critics caution…" Ibid. 724

88. Physicians in no country… See Chapter 10.

88. in Britain for another 3 to 5 years… Alastair Buchan interview 9/7/2009

89. "suffering from the Hawthorne…" e-mail message to JGS: 6/21/2009

89. survey conducted in 2005… Brown et al. (2005)

89. "sparked off controversy…" Lenzer (2004); this article has also appeared under the byline of Owen Dyer.

89. "Imagine you are underneath…" Quoted in Ibid.

90. This analysis of the NINDS… Hacke et al. (2004)

90. Hoffman again brought up… Hoffman and Cooper (2005)

90. "as not designed, however…" Hoffman (2009)

90. "The New Alchemy…" Lenzer (2005)

90. "stop acting as lapdogs…" Ibid.

90. "not from his stroke but…" Lenzer (2008)

90. "So, like many physicians,…" Ibid.

90. "Dr. Hoffman has a brilliant mind…" Ibid.

91. "When myths convince us…" Hoffman and King (2000)

91. In a letter made public... Letter addressed to Dr. Chan and signed by Katherine L. Heilpern, MD (President) and Jill M. Baren, MD (President-elect), dated January 22, 2009. http://www.saem.org/saemdnn/Home/Communities/InterestGroups/NeurologicEmerg/tabid/132/Default.aspxSee also SoRelle (2009).

91. "The time is ripe for a change..." Yu-Feng Yvonne Chan, MD, interview 8/21/2009

91. A movement in favor... NETT: http://nett.umich.edu/nett/welcome;FERNE: http://www.ferne.org/

92. "If you go to a resident-based meeting..." Andy Jagoda interview 8/31/2009

92. "We know that despite our efforts..." McNamara (2009), 340

92. "I believe we need to declare..." Ibid. 339

92. "just empty talk...." Jagoda interview 8/31/200 9136

92. "Because [tPA] is standard of care..." Ibid.

Chapter 7 Money and Brains

95. Genentech's annual report for 1996... See http://www.gene.com/gene/ir/financials/annual-reports/1996/pdf/mrktprod.pdf

95. "for the long-term treatment..." Ibid. 3

95. "The Message is Urgency."... Ibid. 7

95. "recovered with no signs of..." Ibid. 7

95. "I think the company made..." Brott interview 4/16/2007

96. "They initially helped us..." Grotta interview 2/18/2009

96. "told us that stroke..." JAZ/JGS interview 3/7/2007

96. "the driving force to give..." Raab and Bugos (2002), 21

96. "tremendous job of pre-marketing..." Quoted in Pollack (1988)

96. "showed to the physician community..." Raab and Bugos (2002), 26

97. "to see it stall around a..." Heynecker and Hughes (2002), 135

97. "We told them we'd take..." Brott interview 4/16/2007

97. "They didn't think there was going..." William F. Bennett interview 3/11/2008

97. "We didn't have what you would..." Ibid.

99. Until recently, the associated reimbursement... Ibid. 662

100. Reimbursement for doctors... Ibid. 663

100. A code was eventually... Demaerschalk (2007)

100. "You had some hospitals that..." Joseph P. Broderick interview 2/27/2008

100. Susan C. Fagan and a number of NINDS colleagues... Fagan et al. (1998)

101. A recent study by Danish economist... Ehlers et al. (2007)

101. "saved money and saved QALYs."... Susan Fagan interview 4/4/1008

101. Analyses conducted in… Quinn, Dawson, and Lees (2008)

101. "results of economic analysis are…" Ibid. 186

101. In late 2005, pressure on CMS… Demaerschalk (2007)

Chapter 8 Deer in the Headlights

The narrative of Judy Mead's stroke is based on a series of interviews with Don Mead, Eugene Locken, and Annise Spangler together with the transcripts of depositions as noted below.

106. Dr. Khan's neurological exam… Deposition of Sadaf Yasin Khan, MD, Lompoc, California, Friday, February 20, 2009

107. She later said she had given… Ibid. 9

107. She believed she had detected… Ibid. 67

107. "Discussed with Dr. Ente…" Ibid. 120

108. "There is a blockage there…" Don Mead interview 8/16/2009

109. "They booted up the MRIs…" Deposition of Don Mead, January 21, 2009, 104

110. "No, your wife—I saw it…" Mead interview 9/6/2009; also Annise Spangler

110. The Lompoc Community Hospital administration… Mead interview 9/6/2009; also Annise Spangler

111. "legal quagmire…" Weintraub (2006)

111. One of them, written with Liang… Liang, Lew and Zivin (2008)

111. Another went to the *Annals of Emergency Medicine*… Liang and Zivin (2008)

111. "The typical characteristics of a stroke…" Ibid. 161

111. "may not continue in the…" Liang, Lew, and Zivin (2008), 1432

112. First, a "pooled analysis…" Referring to Hacke et al. (2004)

112. nearly 6 in 10 tPA-treated patients… Liang, Lew, and Zivin (2008), 1430

112. study data published in 2004… Saver (2004)

112. a third analysis involved… Liang, Lew, and Zivin (2008), 1431

112. "reasonable degree of medical probability"… Eugene Locken interview 8/15/2009

112. Joined by his step-daughter Gina, Don… Don Mead and Gina Allman, Plaintiffs, vs. Sadaf Yasin Khan, MD; Maria Cecilia Ramos, MD; Philip Ente, MD; Lompoc Healthcare District (Lompoc Valley Medical Center) and Does 1 to 50, inclusive, Defendants. Case No. 1271703. (California) In a 2010 paper… Lees et al. (2010)

113. In his deposition… Deposition of Don Mead, January 21, 2009

113. "not being able to…" Ibid. 17

113. In a 2010 paper… Lees et al. (2010)

113. "If I had turned left at the end of…" Ibid. 27

113. "left leg would withdraw to pain…" Deposition of Sadaf Yasin Khan, MD, Lompoc, California, February 20, 2009, 25

113. "In further notes…" Ibid. 38

114. "certainly a stroke was part of…" Ibid. 36

114. as Dr. Khan claimed in her deposition… Ibid. 40

114. "What I found in this particular…" Locken interview 8/15/2009

114. "custom and practice…" Deposition of Sadaf Yasin Khan, 82

114. "rapidly improving…." Ibid. 90; 84

114. "showing spontaneous movement in the…" Deposition of Philip Ente, MD, San Luis Obispo, California, April 13, 2009, 7

115. "I asked her, 'When the leg is'…" Ibid. 8

115. This interchange was made odd… Deposition of Sadaf Yasin Khan, 38-9

115. "On initial presentation before…" Deposition of Philip Ente, 27

115. "had we given this patient…" Ibid. 16

115. "Citing three articles…" Russell (1997). The articles were cited, but not by title, by Dr. Ente; they were shown as exhibits to JAZ during his deposition.

115. "Must be good,…" Deposition of Justin Allen Zivin, MD, San Diego, California, July 14, 2009, 47

116. "My question to you…." Ibid. 48

116. He could predict: 58%…. Ibid. 116

117. "I don't have any disagreement that…Deposition of Gregory W. Albers, MD, July 28, 2009, 39

117. "I don't think tPA would have…" Ibid. 110

117. "This is what attorneys always…" Locken interview 8/15/2009

117. "when you mix good prognosis…" Deposition of Gregory W. Albers, 125

117. "Mediation is where you search for…" Lockern interview 8/15/2009

118. "You're going to have to show us…" Ibid.

118. A small study that used… Ibid., in reference to Thomalla et al. (2008)

Chapter 9 Call 911, 112, 15…Even 999

120. For the European Union… The two studies referred to are SITS-ISTR (Wahlgran et al. [2008]) and ECASS III (Hacke et al. 2008). Overall, Europe was a late-comer in the use of tPA for stroke. A review article (Branin et al. [2000]) on acute stroke therapy in Europe, which received data from 22 countries, was published at the turn of the century and contains no reference to thrombolysis.

120. "There is a long way to…" Kaste (2007), 241

120. "We cannot give tPA in France…" Didier Leys interview 8/28/2009

121. "Which is not bad…." Ibid.

121. "In Italy it is dependent…" Ibid.

121. "Spain is working well…." Ibid.

121. "If you go more to the eastern…" Ibid.

121. "battle of the clotbusters…" M. O'Donnell (1991)

121. "barefoot doctor…" Ibid. 1260

121. Streptokinase went on… Interviews with Alastair Buchan 9/7/2009 and Kennedy Lees 2/18/2009

122. "There is still relatively poor…" Charles Warlow interview 8/21/2009

122. International Stroke Trial (IST-III)… http://www.dcn.ed.ac.uk/ist3/

122. "creating uncertainty"… Kennedy Lees interview 2/18/2009

122. "Some of it was doubt created…" Ibid.

122. "by about 10 to 15 years…." Buchan interview 9/7/2009

122. "The Canadian system has sort of…" Ibid.

123. "Act   F.A.S.T."   http://www.stroke.org.uk/information/recognising_stroke_with_the_fast_test/index.html

123. "It all started in Europe, and…" Werner Hacke interview 11/4/2009

123. Hacke delivered the first reports… Hacke (1983)

123. ECASS III in particular… Hacke (2008); see also, e.g., Lyden (2008)

123. "You don't have it on…" Hacke interview 11/4/2009

123. That Japan became… Yamaguchi et al. (2006)

124. Implementation of acute stroke… Takenori Yamaguchi interview 3/2/2010

Chapter 10 Persistence of a Most Controversial Drug

125. In the awkward, trademarked… http://www.strokeassociation.org/presenter.jhtml?identifier=3002728

126. just over 1% of… Schumacher et al. (2007)

126. Those numbers would improve a… Bambauer et al (2006)

126. Although the numbers have… The Joint Commission's Certificate of Distinction for Primary Stroke Centers: see http://www.jointcommission.org/CertificationPrograms/PrimaryStrokeCenters/ Known officially since 2007 as the Joint Commission, it is still sometimes referred to as the Joint Commission on Accreditation of Healthcare Organizations (JCAHO).

126. The American Heart Association… Members of the Brain Attack Coalition and the American Heart/Stroke Association initiated talks with the Joint Commission about 2003 that resulted in the certification program for acute ischemic stroke and the establishment of primary stroke centers. Jean Range interview 3/5/2010

127. In cooperation with the Ad Council… See http://www.adcouncil.org/default.aspx?id=59

127. "A lot of people all thought that..." JAZ/JGS interview 2/2/2007

128. By general agreement it was... See, e.g., Donnan (2003).

128. In 2009 people were... Kleindorfer, Khoury, Broderick, et al. (2009)

129. So unexpected was the washout... Zivin (2007); Cheng, Al-Khoury, and Zivin (2004)

129. One article in the journal *Stroke*... Gladstone (2002)

129. In 2006, a review by Jeff Saver... Saver (2006)

131. Julien Bogousslavsky described... Bogousslavsky (2002)

131. Carefully designed by a group... Tilley et al. (1996)

131. "The treatment effect must be huge..." Saver interview 2/19/09

131. Developed only in the late 1980s... Laupacis (1988)

131. Some physicians did not fully... Halvorsen et al (2003)

131. The NINDS Study, wrote Robert C. Solomon... Solomon (2002)

132. As Jeff Saver viewed matters... Saver (2004)

132. "That type of dichotomization was..." Saver interview 2/19/2009

132. "The NNT for 1 additional... Saver (2004), 1068

133. A pioneering randomized trial showed that... See Robertson (1998).

133. James T. Robertson has recalled... Ibid. 2435

134. The American Heart Association... Neale (2009)

134. "We don't have to go into..." Presentation at Stroke 2009: "Phase III Trials of IV Thrombolysis Beyond 3 Hours"

134. Peter Sandercock, explained that... Presentation at Stroke 2009: "Phase III Trials of IV Thrombolysis Beyond 3 Hours"

135. Nancy Edwards, an emergency physician... Presentation at Stroke 2009: "Telemedicine vs. Telephonic Advice for tPA Administration: The Tortoise or the Hare"

135. *Lancet Neurology* had published an article... Meyer et al. (2008)

135. "We know speed, accuracy..." Quoted in Berthold (2009)

135. "I'm zooming in on you..." Presentation: Telemedicine vs. Telephonic Advice for tPA Administration; details confirmed by interview with Meyer 10/21/2009

137. Five years later that figure had... Kleindorfer, Khoury et al. (2009)

137. "In the Cincinnati population,..." Kleindorfer interview 2/18/2009

Chapter 11   Through the Looking Glass

140. "the national and local campaigns..." Kleindorfer, Khourly, et al. (2009), 2505; Lisabeth and Kleindorfer (2009)

140. Target audiences included... Willey, Williams, and Boden-Albala (2009)

140. the nonprofit Goddess Fund... See http://www.thegoddessfund.org/

141. One way to find…. See via the Internet Stroke Center http://www.strokecenter.org/strokecenters.html

141. Every year several hundred… Lloyd-Jones et al. (2010). Online at http://circ.ahajournals.org/cgi/content/full/121/7/e46

142. Laser treatment is one of these… Zivin, Albers, et al. (2009)

143. A fitting conclusion… The narrative that follows is based on interviews with Boris Vern 11/12/2009

Bibliography

Albers, G. W., Bates V. E., Clarke, W. M., Bell, R., Verro, P., & Hamilton, S. A. (2000). Intravenous tissue-type plasminogen activator for treatment of acute stroke: the Standard Treatment with Alteplase to Reverse Stroke (STARS) study. *Journal of the American Medical Association* 283: 1145-50.

Astrup, T., & Permin, P. M. (1947). Fibrinolysis in the animal organism. *Nature* 161: 689-90.

Baker, R. N., Broward JA, Fang HC, Fisher CM, Broch SN, Heyman A, et al. (1962). Anticoagulant therapy in cerebral infarction. Report on cooperative study. *Neurology* 12: 823-35.

Bambauer KZ, Johnston SC, Bambauer DE, & Zivin, J. (2006). Reasons why few patients with acute stroke receive tissue plasminogen activator. *Archives of Neurology* 63: 661-4.

Bazell, R. (1998). *Her2: The Making of Herceptin, a Revolutonary Treatment for Breast Cancer*. New York: Random House.

Bera, R. K. (2009). The story of the Cohen–Boyer patents. *Current Science* 96(6): 760-3.

Berthold, J. (2009). Help from afar. *ACP Internist*. Available at: http://www.acpinternist. org/archives/2009/04/telestroke.htm

Bogousslavsky, J. (2002). Thrombolysis in acute stroke. *British Medical Journal* 313: 640-1.

Brainin, M., Bornstein, N., Boysen, G., & Demarin, V. (2000). Acute neurological stroke care in Europe: results of the European Stroke Care Inventory. *European Journal of Neurology* 7(1): 5-10.

Broderick, J. (1997). Logistics in acute stroke management. *Drugs* 54 (Suppl 3): 109-16.

Brown, D. L., Barsan, W. G., Lisabeth, L. D., Gallery, M. E., & Morgenstern, L. B. (2005). Survey of emergency physicians about recombinant tissue plasminogen activator for acute ischemic stroke. *Annals of Emergency Medicine* 46(1): 56-60.

Brown, M. (1997). *Emergency! True Stories from the Nation's ER*. New York: St. Martin's.

Caplan, L. R. (2009). *Caplan's Stroke: A Clinical Approach*. Philadelphia: Saunders.

Caplan, L. R., Mohr, J. P., Kistler, J. P., & Koroshetz, W. (1997). Should thrombolytic therapy be the first-line treatment for acute ischemic stroke? Thrombolysis—not a panacea for ischemic stroke. *New England Journal of Medicine* 337(18): 1309-13.

Cheng, Y. D., Al-Khoury, L., & Zivin, J. A. (2004). Neuroprotection for ischemic stroke: two decades of success and failure. *NeuroRx* 1(1): 36-45.

Clark, W. M., Wissman, S., Albers G. W., Jhamandas, J. H., Madden, K. P., & Hamilton, S. (1999). Recombinant tissue-type plasminogen activator (Alteplase) for ischemic stroke 3 to 5 hours after symptom onset. The ATLANTIS Study: a randomized controlled trial. Alteplase Thrombolysis for Acute Noninterventional Therapy in Ischemic Stroke. *Journal of the American Medical Association* 282: 2019-26.

Collen, D. (1996). Fibrin-selective thrombolytic therapy for acute myocardial infarction. *Circulation* 93(5): 857-65.

Collen, D., & Lijnen, H. R. (2004). Tissue-type plasminogen activator: a historical perspective and personal account. *Journal of Thrombosis & Haemostasis* 2(4): 541-6.

Cornu, C., Boutitie, F., Candelise, L., Boissel, J. P., Donnan, G. A., Hommel, M., Jaillard, A., & Lees, K. R. (2000). Streptokinase in acute ischemic stroke: an individual patient data meta-Analysis. *Stroke* 31: 1555–60.

Del Zoppo, G. J., Copeland, B. R., Waltz, T. A., Zyroff, J., Plow E. F., & Harker, L. A. (1986). The beneficial effect of intracarotid urokinase on acute stroke in a baboon model. *Stroke* 17(4): 638-43.

Demaerschalk, B. M. (2007). How diagnosis-related group 559 will change the U.S. Medicare cost reimbursement ratio for stroke centers. *Stroke* 38: 1309.

Donnan, G. A., & Davis, S. M. (2001). When is enough enough? *Stroke* 32: 2710-1.

Donnan, G. A., & Davis, S. M. (2003). Controversy: the essence of medical debate. *Stroke* 34: 372-3.

Edwards, L. L. (2007). Using tPA for acute stroke in a rural setting. *Neurology* 68: 292-4.

Ehlers, L., Andersen, G., Clausen, L. B., Bech, M., & Kjølby, M. (2007). Cost-effectiveness of intravenous thrombolysis with alteplase within a 3-hour window after acute ischemic stroke. *Stroke* 38: 85-9.

Ehrenhalt, A. (1996). *The Lost City: Discovering the Forgotten Virtues of Community in the Chicago of the 1950s*. New York: Basic Books.

Fagan, S. C., Morgenstern, L. B., Petitta, A., Ward, R. E., Tilley, B. C., Marler, J. R., Levine, S. R., Broderick, J. P., Kwiatkowski, T. G., Frankel, M., Brott, T. G., & Walker, M.D. (1998). Cost-effectiveness of tissue plasminogen activator for acute ischemic stroke. NINDS rt-PA Stroke Study Group. *Neurology* 50(4): 883-90.

Fields, W. S., & Lemak, N. A. (1989). *A History of Stroke: Its Recognition and Treatment*. New York: Oxford University Press.

Furlan, A. J. (1997). When is thrombolysis justified in patients with acute ischemic stroke? *Stroke* 28: 214-8.

Furlan, A. J. (2000). CVA: reducing the risk of a confused vascular analysis. The Feinberg lecture. *Stroke* 31(6): 1451-6.

Genton, E., Barnett, H. J., Fields, W. S., Gent, M., & Hoak, J. C. (1977). XIV. Cerebral ischemia: the role of thrombosis and of antithrombotic therapy. Study group on antithrombotic therapy. *Stroke* 8(1): 150-75.

Gladstone, D. J., Black, S. E., & Hakim, A. M. (2002). Toward wisdom from failure: lessons from neuroprotective stroke trials and new therapeutic directions. *Stroke* 33: 2123-36.

Goldstein, M. (2008). Remembrance of things past: a summary of the development of cerebrovascular terminology in modern times. *Journal of Stroke & Cerebrovascular Diseases* 17(2): 47-8.

Grotta, J. (1997). Should thrombolytic therapy be the first-line treatment for acute ischemic stroke? t-PA: the best current option for most patients. *New England Journal of Medicine* 337(18): 1310-3.

Grotta, J., & Marler, J. (2007). Intravenous rt-PA: a tenth anniversary reflection. *Surgical Neurology* 68(Suppl 1): S12-6.

Hachinski, V., & Norris, J. W. (1985). *The Acute Stroke*. Philadelphia: F. A. Davis.

Hacke, W., Donnan, G., Fieschi, C., Kaste, M., von Kummer, R., Broderick, J. P., Brott, T., Frankel, M., Grotta, J. C., Haley, E. C. Jr., Kwiatkowski, T., Levine, S. R., Lewandowski, C., Lu, M., Lyden, P., Marler, J. R., Patel, S., Tilley, B. C., Albers, G., Bluhmki, E., Wilhelm, M., & Hamilton, S.; ATLANTIS Trials Investigators; ECASS Trials Investigators; NINDS rt-PA Study Group Investigators. (2004). Association of outcome with early stroke treatment: pooled analysis of ATLANTIS, ECASS, and NINDS rt-PA stroke trials. *Lancet* 363(9411): 768-74.

Hacke, W., Kaste, M., Bluhmki, E., Brozman, M., Dávalos, A., Guidetti, D., Larrue, V., Lees, K. R., Medeghri, Z., Machnig, T., Schneider, D., von Kummer, R., Wahlgren, N., & Toni, D.; ECASS Investigators (2008). Thrombolysis with alteplase 3 to 4.5 hours after acute ischemic stroke. *New England Journal of Medicine* 359(13): 1317-29.

Hacke W., Berg-Dammer, E., & Zeumer, H. (1983). Evoked potential monitoring during acute occlusion of the basilar artery and selective local thrombolytic therapy. *Archiv für Psychiatrie und Nervenkrankheiten* 232(6): 541-8.

Hacke, W., Kaste, M., Fieschi, C., Toni, D., Lesaffre, E., von Kummer, R., Boysen, G., Bluhmki, E., Höxter, G., Mahagne, M. H., et al. (1995). Intravenous thrombolysis with recombinant tissue plasminogen activator for acute hemispheric stroke: the European Cooperative Acute Stroke Study (ECASS). *Journal of the American Medical Association* 274: 1017-25.

Hadler, N. M. (2008). *Worried Sick*. Chapel Hill: University of North Carolina Press.

Haley, E. C. Jr., Lyden, P. D., Johnston, K. C., & Hemmen, T. M.; TNK in Stroke Investigators. (2005). A pilot dose-escalation safety study of tenecteplase in acute ischemic stroke. *Stroke* 36: 207-12.

Hall, E. T. (1976). *Beyond Culture*. Garden City, NY: Anchor Press.

Hall, S. S. (1987). *Invisible Frontiers: The Race to Synthesize a Human Gene*. New York: Atlantic Monthly Press.

Halvorsen P. A., Kristiansen I. S., Aasland O. G., Førde O. H., (2003) 'Medical doctors' perception of the "number needed to treat" (NNT). *Scand J Prim Health Care* 21(3): 162-6.

Hass, W. K. (1983). The cerebral ischemic cascade. *Neurology Clinics* 1(1): 345-53.

Hay, J. W. (2005). The application of cost-effectiveness and cost-benefit analysis to pharmaceuticals. In: Santoro, M. A., & Gorrie, T. M., eds. *Ethics and the Pharmaceutical Industry*. New York: Cambridge University Press, pp. 225-47.

Henig, R. M. (1997). *The People's Health*. Washington, DC: Joseph Henry Press.

Heyneker, H. L., & Hughes, S. S. (2002). Molecular geneticist at UCSF and Genentech, entrepreneur in biotechnology. Program in the History of the Biological Sciences and Biotechnology, Regional Oral History Office, The Bancroft Library, University of California, Berkeley. Available at: http://content.cdlib.org/ark:/13030/hb0n39n481/?query=heyneker&brand=calisphere.

Hoffman, J. (2000). Should physicians give tPA to patients with acute ischemic stroke? Against: and just what is the emperor of stroke wearing? *Western Journal of Medicine* 173(3): 149-50.

Hoffman, J. (2009). Acute ischemic stroke—update 2009. Course syllabus for emergency medicine & acute care: a critical appraisal. Key West, FL.

Hoffman, J. R. (2003). Tissue plasminogen activator (tPA) for acute ischaemic stroke: why so much has been made of so little. *Medical Journal of Australia* 179(7): 333-4.

Hoffman, J. R., & King, K. C. (2000). Myths and medicine. *Western Journal of Medicine* 172(3): 208.

Hoffman, J. R., & Cooper, R. J. (2005). Stroke thrombolysis: we need new data, not more reviews. *Lancet* 4(4): 204-5.

Horowitz, S. H. (1998). Thrombolytic therapy in acute stroke: neurologists, get off your hands! *Archives of Neurology* 55(2): 155-7.

Ingall, T. J., O'Fallon, W. M., Asplund, K., Goldfrank, L. R., Hertzberg, V. S., Louis, T. A., & Christianson, T. J. (2004). Findings from the reanalysis of the NINDS tissue plasminogen activator for acute ischemic stroke treatment trial. *Stroke* 35(10): 2418-24.

Jones, T. H., Morawetz, R. B., Crowell, R. M., Marcoux, F. W., FitzGibbon, S. J., DeGirolami, U., & Ojemann, R. G. (1981). Thresholds of focal cerebral ischemia in awake monkeys. *Journal of Neurosurgery* 51: 773-82.

Katzan, I. L., Hammer, M. D., Furlan, A. J., Hixson, E. D., & Nadzam, D. M. (2003). Quality improvement and tissue-type plasminogen activator for acute ischemic stroke: a Cleveland update. *Stroke* 34: 799-800.

Katzan, I. L., Sila, C. A. & Furlan, A. J. (2001). Community use of intravenous tissue plasminogen activator for acute stroke: results of the brain matters stroke management survey. *Stroke* 32(4): 861-5.

Katzan, I. L., Furlan, A. J., Lloyd, L. E., Frank, J. I., Harper, D. L., Hinchey, J. A., Hammel, J. P., Qu, A., & Sila, C. A. (2000). Use of tissue-type plasminogen activator for acute ischemic stroke: the Cleveland area experience. *Journal of the American Medical Association* 283: 1151-8.

Kleid, D. G., & Hughes, S. S. (2002). Scientist and patent agent at Genentech. Program in the History of the Biological Sciences and Biotechnology, Regional Oral History

Office, The Bancroft Library, University of California, Berkeley. Available at: http://content.cdlib.org/view?docId=hb1t1n98fg&doc.view=frames&chunk.id=div00144&toc.depth=1&toc.id=div00143&brand=oac.

Kleindorfer, D., Khoury, J., Broderick, J. P., Rademacher, E., Woo, D., Flaherty, M. L., Alwell, K., Moomaw, C. J., Schneider, A., Pancioli, A., Miller, R., & Kissela, B. M. (2009). Temporal trends in public awareness of stroke: warning signs, risk factors, and treatment. *Stroke* 40(7): 2502-6.

Kleindorfer, D., Xu, Y., Moomaw, C. J., Khatri, P., Adeoye, O., & Hornung, R. (2009). U.S. geographic distribution of rt-PA utilization by hospital for acute ischemic stroke. *Stroke* 40(11): 3580-4.

Kwiatkowski, T. G., Libman, R. B., Frankel, M., Tilley, B. C., Morgenstern, L. B., Lu, M., Broderick, J. P., Lewandowski, C. A., Marler, J. R., Levine, S. R., & Brott, T. (1999). Effects of tissue plasminogen activator for acute ischemic stroke at one year. National Institute of Neurological Disorders and Stroke Recombinant Tissue Plasminogen Activator Stroke Study Group. *New England Journal of Medicine* 340(23): 1781-7.

Lattimore, S. U., Chalela, J., Davis, L., DeGraba, T., Ezzeddine, M., Haymore, J., Nyquist, P., Baird, A. E., Hallenbeck, J., & Warach, S. (2003). Impact of establishing a primary stroke center at a community hospital on the use of thrombolytic therapy: the NINDS Suburban Hospital Stroke Center experience. *Stroke* 34: e55-7.

Laupacis, A., Sackett, D. L., & Roberts, R. S. (1988). An assessment of clinically useful measures of the consequences of treatment. *New England Journal of Medicine* 318(26): 1728-33.

Le Fanu, J. (1999). *The Rise and Fall of Modern Medicine*. London: Little, Brown.

Kennedy R. Lees, Bluhmki E. von Kummer R., et al., for the ECASS, ATLANTIS, NINDS and EPITHET rt-PA Study Group Investigators. (2010). Time to treatment with intravenous alteplase and outcome in stroke: an updated pooled analysis of ECASS, ATLANTIS, NINDS, and EPITHET trials *Lancet* 375(9727):1695-1703.

Lenzer, J. (2002). Alteplase for stroke: money and optimistic claims buttress the brain attack campaign. *British Medical Journal* 324(7339): 723-9.

Lenzer, J. (2004). Reanalysis of alteplase for stroke stirs controversy. *British Medical Journal* 329: 820.

Lenzer, J. (2005). The new alchemy: Mixing doctors and journalists to spin gold. Healthy Skepticism International News. Available at: http://www.healthyskepticism.org/global/news/int/hsin2005-04/

Lenzer, J. (2008). Wonder drugs that can kill. *Discover Magazine*. Available at: http://discovermagazine.com/2008/jul/20-wonder-drugs-that-can-kill.

Liang, B. A., & Zivin, J. A. (2008). Empirical characteristics of litigation involving tissue plasminogen activator and ischemic stroke. *Annals of Emergency Medicine* 52(2): 160-4.

Liang, B. A., Lew, R., & Zivin, J. A. (2008). Review of tissue plasminogen activator, ischemic stroke, and potential legal issues. *Archives of Neurology* 65(11): 1429-33.

Lindley, R. I. (2001). Further randomized controlled trials of tissue plasminogen activator within 3 hours are required. *Stroke* 32: 2708-9.

Lingen, H., ed. (2008). *Désiré Collen: An Anthology of Scientific Collaborations, Compiled at the Occasion of his 65th Birthday*. Leuven, Belgium [printed privately].

Lisabeth, L. D., & Kleindorfer, D. (2009). Stroke literacy in high-risk populations: a call for action. *Stroke* 73(23): 1950-6.

Lloyd-Jones, D., Adams, R. J., Brown, T. M., Carnethon, M., Dai, S., De Simone, G., Ferguson, T. B., Ford, E., Furie, K., Gillespie, C., Go, A., Greenlund, K., Haase, N., Hailpern, S., Ho, P. M., Howard, V., Kissela, B., Kittner, S., Lackland, D., Lisabeth, L., Marelli, A., McDermott, M. M., Meigs, J., Mozaffarian, D., Mussolino, M., Nichol, G., Roger, V. L., Rosamond, W., Sacco, R., Sorlie, P., Stafford, R., Thom, T., Wasserthiel-Smoller, S., Wong, N. D., & Wylie-Rosett, J. (2010). Executive summary: heart disease and stroke statistics—2010 update: a report from the American Heart Association. *Circulation* 121(7): 948-54.

Lyden, P. (2008). Thrombolytic therapy for acute stroke—not a moment to lose. *New England Journal of Medicine* 359(13): 1395.

Lyden, P. D. (2001). Further randomized controlled trials of tPA within 3 hours are required—NOT! *Stroke* 32: 2209-10.

Lyden, P. D., & Zivin, J. A. (1993). Hemorrhagic transformation after cerebral ischemia: mechanisms and incidence. *Cerebrovascular and Brain Metabolism Reviews* 5(1): 1-16.

Lyden, P. D., Madden K. P., Clark, W. M., Sasse, K. C., & Zivin, J. A. (1990). Incidence of cerebral hemorrhage after treatment with tissue plasminogen activator or streptokinase following embolic stroke in rabbits. *Stroke* 21(11): 1589-93.

Marler, J. R. (2002). NINDS-sponsored clinical trials in stroke: past, present, and future. *Stroke* 33(1): 311-2.

Marler, J. R., Tilley, B. C., Lu, M., Brott, T. G., Lyden, P. C., Grotta, J. C., Broderick, J. P., Levine, S. R., Frankel, M. P., Horowitz, S. H., Haley, E. C. Jr., Lewandowski, C. A., & Kwiatkowski, T. P. (2000). Early stroke treatment associated with better outcome: the NINDS rt-PA stroke study. *Neurology* 55(11): 1649-55.

Maroo, A., & Topol, E. J. (2004). The early history and development of thrombolysis in acute myocardial infarction. *Journal of Thrombosis & Haemostasis* 2(11): 1867-70.

Marsa, L. (1997). *Prescription for Profits*. New York: Scribner.

Mattews, D., & McPherson, K. (1987). Doctors' ignorance of statistics. *British Medical Journal* 294: 856-7.

McElroy, C. R., & Hoffman, J. R. (1981). Still more HAFE. *Western Journal of Medicine* 134(6): 546.

McNamara, R. (2009). Thrombolysis in stroke: still not ready for community hospital use by emergency physicians. *Annals of Emergency Medicine* 54(3): 339-41.

Meyer, B. C., Raman, R., Hemmen, T., Obler, R., Zivin, J. A., Rao, R., Thomas, R. G., & Lyden, P. D. (2008). Efficacy of site-independent telemedicine in the STRokE DOC trial: a randomised, blinded, prospective study. *Lancet Neurology* 7(9): 1787-95.

Meyer, J. S., Gilroy, J., Barnhart, M. E., & Johnson, J. F. (1965). Therapeutic thrombolysis in cerebral thromboembolism: randomized evaluation of intravenous streptokinase. In: Millikan, C. H., Siekert, R. G., & Whisnant, J. P., eds., *Cerebral Vascular Diseases*, Fourth Princeton Conference. New York: Grune and Stratton, 1965, pp. 200-13.

Miller, Henry I. (1997). *Policy Controversy in Biotechnology: An Insider's View*. Austin, TX.: R.G. Landes Company and Academic Press.

Mohr, J. P. (2000). Thrombolytic therapy for ischemic stroke. *Journal of the American Medical Association* 283: 1189-91.

Montgomery, M. R. (Aug. 21, 1983). *The selling of science*. Boston Globe.

Mueller, C., & Scheidt, S. (1994). History of drugs for thrombotic disease. *Circulation* 89(1): 432-49.

Neale, T. (2009). Post-stroke thrombolysis window expanded to 4.5 hours. *MedPage Today*. Available at: http://www.medpagetoday.com/Cardiology/Strokes/14414

NINDS rt-PA Stroke Study Group. (1995). Tissue plasminogen activator for acute ischemic stroke. *New England Journal of Medicine* 333: 1581-7.

O'Donnell, M. (1991). Battle of the clotbusters. *British Medical Journal* 302(6787): 2159-61.

Osler, W. (1908). *Counsels and Ideals from the Writings of William Osler*. Boston: Houghton Mifflin.

Owen, C. A. (2001). *A History of Blood Coagulation*. Rochester, Minn.: Mayo Foundation for Medical Education and Research.

Pennica, D., Holmes, W. E., Kohr, W. J., Harkins, R. N., Vehar, G. A., Ward, C. A., Bennett, W. F., Yelverton, E., Seeburg, P. H., Heyneker, H. L., Goeddel, D. V., & Collen, D. (1983). Cloning and expression of human tissue-type plasminogen activator cDNA in *E. coli*. *Nature* 301(5897): 214-21.

Plum, F. (1983). What causes infarction in ischemic brain? The Robert Wartenberg Lecture. *Neurology* 33(2): 222-33.

Pollack, A. (Jan. 5, 1988). Fast start for bioengineered drug. *New York Times*.

Porter, R. (1997). *The Greatest Benefit to Mankind: A Medical History of Humanity*. New York: W. W. Norton.

Quinn, T. J., Dawson, J., & Lees, K. R. (2008). Past, present and future of alteplase for acute ischemic stroke. *Expert Review of Neurotherapeutics* 8(2): 181-92.

Raab, G. K., & B., Glenn E. (2002). CEO at Genentech 1990–1995. Program in the History of the Biological Sciences and Biotechnology, Regional Oral History Office, The Bancroft Library, University of California, Berkeley. Available at:

Raichle, M. E. (1982). The pathophysiology of brain ischemia and infarction. *Clinical Neurosurgery* 29: 379-89.

Riggs, J. E. (1996). Tissue-type plasminogen activator should not be used in acute ischemic stroke. *Archives of Neurology* 53(12): 1306-8.

Rijken, D. C., & Collen, D. (1981). Purification and characterization of the plasminogen activator secreted by human melanoma cells in culture. *Journal of Biological Chemistry* 256(13): 7035-41.

Rijken, D. C., Hoylaerts, M., & Collen D. (1982). Fibrinolytic properties of one-chain and two-chain human extrinsic (tissue-type) plasminogen activator. *Journal of Biological Chemistry* 257(6): 2920-25.

Robbins-Roth, C. (2000). *From Alchemy to IPO*. New York: Basic Books.

Roberts, W. C. (1972). Coronary arteries in fatal acute myocardial infarction. *Circulation* 45(1): 215-30.

Robertson, J. T. (1998). Carotid endarterectomy: a saga of clinical science, personalities, and evolving technology. *Stroke* 29(2435): 2441.

Rozenthul-Sorokin, N., Ronen, R., Tamir, A., Geva, H., & Eldar, R. (1996). Stroke in the young in Israel: incidence and outcomes. *Stroke* 27: 838-41.

Russell, E. (1997). Diagnosis of hyperacute ischemic infarct with CT: key to improved clinical outcome after intravenous thrombolysis? *Radiology* 205(174): 315-8.

Saver, J. (2004). Number needed to treat estimates incorporating effects over the entire range of clinical outcomes. *Archives of Neurology* 204(61): 1066-70.

Saver, J. L. (2006). Time is brain—quantified. *Stroke* 37: 263-6.

Scheck, A. (2003). Making a difference as the odd man out. *Emergency Medicine News* 25(7): 4. Available at: http://journals.lww.com/em-news/Fulltext/2003/07000/Making_a_Difference_as_the_Odd_Man_Out.4.aspx

Schiller, F. (1970). Concepts of stroke before and after Virchow. *Medical History* 14(2): 115-31.

Schumacher, H. C., Bateman, B. T., Boden-Albala, B., Berman, M. F., Mohr, J. P., Sacco, R. L., & Pile-Spellman, J. (2007). Use of thrombolysis in acute ischemic stroke: analysis of the Nationwide Inpatient Sample 1999 to 2004. *Annals of Emergency Medicine* 50(2): 99-107.

Sherry, S. (1989). The origin of thrombolytic therapy. *Journal of the American College of Cardiology* 14(4): 1085-92.

Sherry, S. (1992). *Reflections and Reminiscences of an Academic Physician.* Malvern, PA: Lea & Febiger.

Sikri, N., & Bardia, A. (2007). A history of streptokinase use in acute myocardial infarction. *Texas Heart Institute Journal* 34(3): 318-27.

Simmons, J. G. (2002). *Doctors and Discoveries: Lives That Created Today's Medicine.* Boston: Houghton Mifflin.

Sobel, B., Collen, D., & Grossbard, E., eds. (1987). *Tissue Plasminogen Activator in Thrombolytic Therapy.* Chicago: Marcel Dekker.

Solomon, R. C. (2002). Alteplase for stroke. Financial information is needed to ensure objectivity. *British Medical Journal* 324(7353): 1582.

SoRelle, R. (2009). Rethinking tPA for stroke. *Emergency Medicine News* 31(8): 24-5.

Starr, P. (1982). *The Social Transformation of American Medicine.* New York: Basic Books.

Stefanovich, V., ed. (1982). *Stroke: Animal Models.* Advances in Bioscience. New York: Pergamon Press.

Thomalla, G., Kruetzelmann, A., Siemonsen, S., Gerloff, C., Rosenkranz, M., Röther, J., & Fiehler, J. (2008). Clinical and tissue response to intravenous thrombolysis in tandem internal carotid artery/middle cerebral artery occlusion. *Stroke* 39: 1616-8.

Tilley, B. C., Lyden, P. D., Brott, T. G., Lu, M., Levine, S. R., & Welch, K. M. (1997). Total quality improvement method for reduction of delays between emergency department admission and treatment of acute ischemic stroke. The National Institute of Neurological Disorders and Stroke rt-PA Stroke Study Group. *Archives of Neurology* 54(12): 1466-74.

Tilley, B. C., Marler, J., Geller, N. L., Lu, M., Legler, J., Brott, T., Lyden, P., & Grotta, J. (1996). Use of a global test for multiple outcomes in stroke trials with application to the National Institute of Neurological Disorders and Stroke t-PA Stroke Trial. *Stroke* 27: 2136-42.

Virchow, R., ed. (1958). *Disease, Life and Man: Selected Essays by Rudolf Virchow.* Stanford Studies in the Medical Sciences 9. Stanford, CA.: Stanford University Press.

Virchow, R. (1997). *Thrombosis and embolie (1846-1856).* Canton, MA: Science History Publications.

Wahlgren, N., Ahmed, N., Dávalos, A., Hacke, W., Millán, M., Muir, K., Roine, R. O., Toni, D., & Lees, K. R.; SITS investigators. (2008). Thrombolysis with alteplase 3-4.5 h after acute ischaemic stroke (SITS-ISTR). *Lancet* 372(9646): 1303-9.

Weintraub, J. (2006). Thrombolysis (tissue plasminogen activator) in stroke: a medicolegal quagmire. *Stroke* 37: 1917-22.

Weisse, A. B. (2006). The elusive clot: the controversy over coronary thrombosis in myocardial infarction. *Journal of the History of Medicine & Allied Sciences* 61(1): 66-78.

West, C., & Ficalora, R. D. (2007). Clinician attitudes toward biostatistics. *Mayo Clinic Proceedings* 82(12): 1578-9.

Willey, J. Z., William, O., & Boden-Albala, B. (2009). Stroke literacy in Central Harlem: a high-risk stroke population. *Neurology* 73(23): 1940-1.

Yamaguchi, T., Mori, E., Minematsu, K., Nakagawara, J., Hashi, K., Saito, I., & Shinohara, Y.; Japan Alteplase Clinical Trial (J-ACT) Group. (2006). Alteplase at 0.6 mg/kg for acute ischemic stroke within 3 hours of onset: Japan Alteplase Clinical Trial (J-ACT). *Stroke* 37(7): 1810-5.

Zink, B. J. (2005). *Anyone, Anything, Anytime: A History of Emergency Medicine.* Philadelphia: Mosby.

Zivin, J. A. (1998). Factors determining the therapeutic window for stroke. *Neurology* 50(3): 599-603.

Zivin, J. A. (2007). Clinical trials of neuroprotective therapies. *Stroke* 38(2 Suppl): 791-3.

Zivin, J. A., Albers, G. W., Bornstein, N., Chippendale, T., Dahlof, B., Devlin, T., Fisher, M., Hacke, W., Holt, W. Ilic, S., Kasner, S. Lew, R., Nash, M., Perez, J., Rymer, M., Schellinger, P., Schneider, D., Schwab, S., Veltkamp, R., Walker, M., Streeter, J. NeuroThera Effectiveness and Safety Trial-2 Investigators. (2009). Effectiveness and safety of transcranial laser therapy for acute ischemic stroke. *Stroke* 40(4): 1359-64.

Zivin, J. A., & Bartko, J. J. (1976). Statistics for disinterested scientists. *Life Sciences* 18: 15-26.

Zivin, J. A., DeGirolami, U., & Hurwitz, E. L. (1982). Spectrum of neurological deficits in experimental CNS ischemia. A quantitative study. *Archives of Neurology* 39(7): 408-12.

Zivin, J. A., Fisher, M., DeGirolami, U., Hemenway, C. C. & Stashak, J. A. (1985). Tissue plasminogen activator reduces neurological damage after cerebral embolism. *Science* 230(4731): 1289-92.

Zivin, J. A., & Waud, D. R. (1982). How to analyze binding, enzyme and uptake data: the simplest case, a single phase. *Life Sciences* 30(17): 1407-22.

Zivin, J. A., & Waud, D. R. (1983). A precise and sensitive method for measurement of spinal cord blood flow. *Brain Research* 258(2): 197-200.

Zivin, J. A., & Waud, D. R. (1992). Quantal bioassay and stroke. *Stroke* 23(5): 767-73.

Index